The New High Protein Diet

**Dr Charles Clark
and Maureen Clark**

Vermilion
LONDON

13 15 14

First published in 2002 by Vermilion
This new edition published in 2007 by Vermilion, an imprint of Ebury Publishing

A Random House Group Company

The Random House Group Limited Reg. No. 954009

Addresses for companies within the Random House Group can be found at
www.randomhouse.co.uk

A CIP catalogue record for this book is available from the British Library

The Random House Group Limited supports The Forest Stewardship
Council® (FSC®), the leading international forest certification organisation.
All our titles that are printed on Greenpeace approved FSC® certified paper
carry the FSC® logo. Our paper procurement policy can be found at:
www.randomhouse.co.uk/environment

Printed in the UK by CPI Cox & Wyman, Reading, RG1 8EX

ISBN 9780091917333

Copies are available at special rates for bulk orders. Contact the sales development team
on 020 7840 8487 or visit www.booksforpromotions.co.uk for more information.

The advice offered in this book is not intended to be a substitute for the advice
and counsel of your personal physician. Always consult a medical practitioner
before embarking on a diet, or a course of exercise. Neither the authors nor the
publisher can be held responsible for any loss or claim arising out of the use,
or misuse, of the suggestions made, or the failure to take medical advice.

To buy books by your favourite authors and register for offers, visit www.randomhouse.co.uk

The New High Protein Diet

Contents

Acknowledgements

I would like to thank my wife for her patience, understanding, support and considerable advice, without which the book would not have been possible; my son, David, for his occasional patience and understanding; and my daughter, Heather, for her total lack of patience with her father, with the result that life is many things but never boring!

Preface

The New High Protein Diet will change your life. Not only will you lose weight quickly, easily and painlessly, you will also become much healthier with more energy than you have enjoyed for years.

How can we be so certain? Simply because this diet is based on medical principles, not just an alternative exotic method of starving yourself (which is the basis of many diets). On this system, you will enjoy copious quantities of delicious foods which will medically programme your body to burn fat.

The diet has been refined over several years at our private clinic in Devonshire Place in the West End of London. The concepts were first published in the initial edition of this book in 2002, which became an instant bestseller. Since then, we have refined the diet to incorporate the experiences of many of our patients.

The single and the most important point to realise is that dieting has major medical effects on your body apart from just making you look slimmer! As many people know to their cost, simply starving yourself by one method or another may cause weight loss in the early stages, but the weight always piles back on again later. In this system, because you are actually changing your body's hormones to make you burn the fat, the weight simply does not reappear. You will reconfigure your metabolism back to a healthy, slim option. In other words, you will return to the shape you should be naturally, not the shape your diet has given you!

Most people simply want to get on with it, lose weight and feel better and so that is exactly what we are going to do. For those of you who have an interest in understanding exactly how the diet works medically, this is explained later in chapter 2.

For everyone else, let's begin now!

PART I

The New High Protein Diet

If you're overweight, this diet will help you to lose weight quickly, easily and painlessly, and – providing you keep to some very simple guidelines – the weight will not return. Part I of the book explains the basic principles of the diet. It is really essential to read this because when you *understand* the problem it's much easier to solve. And being overweight *is* a medical problem, it's *not* just a question of eating too much, which is the usual explanation given (and which is completely incorrect). It's an imbalance of hormones; in fact, our present high-carbohydrate diet actually stimulates certain hormones to deposit fat. Part I of the book will explain how you can easily *reverse* this process, making the hormones *remove* your body fat preferentially, *despite enjoying a high-calorie diet.* You will be able to eat delicious foods and never be hungry, whilst losing weight at the safest rate for the human body. And you will probably be eating the most nutritious food in your life, as this diet is specially designed to incorporate all of the essential nutrition for health – unlike many other diets. The New High Protein Diet is really a way of life, rather than a diet, in which you re-programme your body to lose weight, and the hormones do the work for you. And the way you re-programme the system is simply by eating certain combinations of healthy foods and avoiding others. It really is that simple. With the correct advice, anyone can lose weight easily and painlessly.

Chapter 1   How *not* to diet

The reason I am explaining how not to diet is that most people have being going about losing weight in the wrong way for years, and I am firmly of the opinion that to lose weight successfully you need to understand why previous diets have failed and why this new diet *will* work.

Studies have shown that less than 5 per cent of people are successful in permanently losing weight on a diet. To put this another way, 95 per cent of dieters fail to lose weight for any significant period of time – most eventually gaining more weight than they had before they started to diet. As all of these people have a real desire to be slimmer, they try another diet, and another one, and so it goes on. And as all of them are serious dieters, a billion-dollar industry develops to service their needs, which is self-sustaining as 95 per cent of the diets fail. This is not intended as a criticism of the diet industry; on the contrary, being slimmer is undoubtedly healthier for most individuals (apart from those with an unrealistic self-image) and therefore a slimmer, healthier body is definitely to be encouraged.

Where most diets go wrong

The problem with the majority of diets is that, without superhuman willpower, the dieter cannot sustain the regime.

And when (not 'if') the diet fails, we are convinced it must be our fault, because, after all, it can't take much willpower to achieve, as we have constant reminders in slimming magazines of 'ordinary' (usually grossly overweight) people who apparently slimmed from 25 to 10 stones without any difficulty at all. So now not only are we unhappy about our weight and appearance, but we are also guilty about our abject failure to lose the fat. What can be so difficult when we have detailed instructions from eminent experts – or even better, the advice of celebrity dieters who seem to lose weight with no problem at all? Of course, the benefits of unlimited free time and money to spend on improving their physical appearance may contribute to their success!

Let us deal with each of these points in turn, because if we can't clear up the mental problem, the physical problem will remain. Most importantly, you have nothing to feel guilty about! You are not a failure, and you are not wrong. The diets are virtually unworkable for almost everybody. How can I be so certain? Simple. Remember I said that current diets failed to achieve sustained weight loss in 95 per cent of cases? As an experienced medical researcher, I can assure you that if an event occurs in 95 per cent of the population, it is considered normal by scientists, and if it occurs in 5 per cent of the population, it is considered abnormal. So, without any doubt, to succeed on present diets is definitely abnormal in scientific terms. In other words, *you* are normal, it's the diet that's not!

How can this be? We are bombarded with constant information regarding the need to reduce our calories; consume less fat, red meat and eggs; eat more vegetables and fruit, and so on. The list is seemingly endless, and we are told that if we do this we will be slimmer and healthier. This is true up to a point, but the problem is that for the majority of people it is a very difficult eating pattern to implement – and worse, it will *not* cause loss of body fat in the majority of circumstances.

Loss of fat medically involves adjusting the *balance* of the various food groups in the diet, not just reducing calories. Unfortunately, loss of body fat is not a simple equation whereby if you reduce your intake of food, you will inevitably lose fat. You won't. All experienced dieters will be familiar with the shock and anger of staring at the non-moving bathroom scales, even though they have eaten virtually nothing. It is balance, not quantity, that makes a diet work. And this makes life much easier for everyone, as you can easily keep to the diet when you find food satisfying, and you feel well, especially when there are no restrictions on the quantities of many tasty foods.

In many instances, when you reduce your intake of food, you lose body protein (especially muscle). So while your body shape may appear smaller, and your waist measurement may decrease, *the amount of body fat remains virtually the same*. What's more, as the underlying layer of body fat is only slightly reduced, when you relinquish your starvation diet and resume eating (even moderately), the body proteins are the first to be reformed by the body, so you rapidly increase in weight (and girth), because protein is twice as heavy as fat. The classic failed diet! So you see, *you* didn't fail: the diet was doomed to failure from the start.

So we arrive at the next obvious question: why bother? If all diets are doomed to failure (or involve intense pain and suffering), there doesn't appear to be much point. Well there is! First, all diets are not doomed to failure: it is only the way in which the diet is *applied* that is unworkable. And second, I can assure you that you will *definitely* lose body fat (not just weight, but actually the fat that you really want to lose) on this diet – easily, painlessly, with little effort or expense, and almost enjoyably. This seems too good to be true, but it is true, as you will see. As an experienced Consultant Surgeon, I am not given to exaggeration; just the facts, pure and simple.

A diet that works

But first of all it is essential to explain the basics of dieting in simple, straightforward terms. Having practised medicine for over twenty years, I am sure that the only way to achieve success in any form of treatment is for patients to be fully informed about their conditions. And let us be perfectly clear about this: being overweight *is* a medical condition, and should be treated as such. Apart from the possible physical problems of obesity (hypertension, heart disease, diabetes, arthritis), the mental distress must be taken seriously: if we are unhappy, our stress levels increase exponentially, and that is a real problem for our ultimate health and well-being.

To the facts of nutrition. Be sure to read this section carefully – it is quite simple to understand – because if you don't fully grasp the principles of the diet, you won't get it right. The first point to make is that you won't be counting calories any more. You are going to adhere to certain rules in choosing foods, which will enable the fat to be 'burned off' (a term I dislike, but it conveys the meaning excellently) by the body. So you will have immense freedom to choose a wide variety of foods *in virtually unlimited quantities*. For the first time, you will eat well while dieting. I know this sounds like some 'never to be repeated offer' on television, but it is based on established medical principles, and does work.

You've probably read some of the following facts before (and almost certainly if you are an experienced dieter) but please read them again, because the subsequent paragraphs will definitely be new to most readers, and form the basis of the diet. Once you understand the principles, you will be able to apply them easily – and successfully.

As most people know, there are five basic food groups that we require: carbohydrates, fats, proteins, vitamins and minerals. The first three (carbohydrates, fats and proteins) give us energy; proteins also provide amino acids, the building blocks of the body. Vitamins and minerals are absolutely essential for the efficient maintenance of body functions (like chemical reactions), but vitamins and minerals *do not* provide energy, and therefore – provided we ensure our diet is not deficient in these essential elements – vitamins and minerals are not part of the weight-loss equation. So, we are left with carbohydrates, fats and protein. The secret of burning body fat lies in the relative proportion of these constituents in the diet.

There are three golden rules that you must understand to diet effectively:

1. Your body does not work like a machine

What does this mean? Let me explain – because this is the reason for the failure of low-calorie diets. The way that scientists determine the energy content (or 'calories') of any given food is literally to burn the food in an instrument, like a type of mini-oven that measures the heat produced. Heat is the way in which energy is 'released' when a material burns, and we give the food a 'caloric content' depending on how much heat is generated. For example, 1 gram of fat produces about 9 calories, whereas 1 gram of carbohydrate or protein produces about 4 calories. Seems fairly simple. On this basis, you might reasonably assume that fat in your diet (as it has twice as many calories as protein or carbohydrate) has twice as much risk of being deposited as fat in your body.

In fact this is wrong. The human body does not function like a machine, and it does not burn food in the same way as a laboratory instrument, so the simple calculation of calories based upon the relative amounts of carbohydrates, proteins and fats is fundamentally flawed. As you will see, by applying medical principles to the way your body processes food, you will be able to eat *more* calories than someone on a low-calorie diet, and yet *you* will lose body fat and they will not. The absorption of food in the gut depends upon a complex series of interactions, which means that by varying the composition of your food, you can eat far more calories (and calories of tasty foods rather than the usual tasteless foods) and lose weight, while someone else may eat fewer calories without losing any weight. Incredible, but true! Now you may begin to see why so many years are wasted counting calories and yet not losing weight – or fat.

2. Fats in your diet do not necessarily cause weight gain

In other words, although fat has double the calorie content of carbohydrate or protein, it does not necessarily cause you to put on twice as much weight. If your diet is properly balanced, you can include a moderate (not excessive) amount of fat in your diet *and actually lose weight.* Once again, this is based upon the fact that the body does not function simply as a machine. This is not intended to encourage you to consume excessive amounts of fats, but rather to eat 'healthy' fats in moderation. In association with the remainder of the programme, you will then lose far more weight (and especially fat) than you ever did counting calories – and with very little effort, you will keep the weight off.

Remember, certain fats are essential components of the human body. (No, I don't mean the bulges over your tummy and hips; we'll get rid of those.) Essential fats make up the outer coating of nerve cells and form the basis of many hormones in the body – including the sex hormones. We need these lipids (a medical term for fats), but not the fat cells deposited in all the wrong places. So you can see that some fats are absolutely essential for a healthy body. You can eat certain fats in your diet, and at the same time remove the unsightly bulges of storage fat around your waist and hips, as this diet will clearly demonstrate. In other words, not all fats are bad.

3. You can programme your body to burn excess body fat instead of dietary calories

This is the most amazing statement of all – the 'Holy Grail' for all dieters. You can programme your body to burn its own fat – especially from the waist and hip region – in preference to the food you consume. In other words, you can have your figurative cake, and eat it.

How can this be possible? Like most of medicine, it's actually very simple, as I'll explain in the next chapter. This information forms the basis of everything that follows. Please take the time to understand it, because you do have to follow the rules of the diet exactly for it to be successful. Once you understand the principles, you will be able to keep to the diet easily, and then you can proceed to eat your way to losing fat.

Chapter 2

How the New High Protein Diet works

To understand the way in which this diet effectively 'burns' excess body fat, we must first of all examine the three main energy foods in our diet and, in particular, their effects on the body when they are digested and absorbed.

The carbohydrate cycle

Carbohydrates are – in simple terms – sugars and starches. They are absorbed from the digestive tract reasonably quickly, which is the reason why we get a rapid energy boost from a bar of chocolate or a pastry. But – and this is the important part – when our blood sugar levels go up, a hormone called insulin is released, which then starts to lower the blood sugar level very quickly. When the sugar level in our blood goes down rapidly, we feel weak and faint ('hypoglycaemia' is medicalspeak for low blood sugar), so we have another sweet food to boost our sugar level. Again, we feel better for a while, and then insulin kicks in to lower our blood sugar and make us feel weak once more. And so the cycle goes on. Most people associate insulin with diabetes, in which there is a problem with insulin production, but actually insulin is an essential hormone in everyone. Your body simply can't cope with too much sugar in the diet.

Every dieter reading this chapter has probably experienced these symptoms. Even worse than the constant ups and downs in energy levels are the difficult mood swings that accompany the energy fluctuations. And every time we have another cake or chocolate – which we really must have or suffer the discomfort of low blood sugar, which nobody can ignore I can assure you – the pounds pile on.

The carbohydrate cycle

Eating refined carbohydrates → More insulin → Lower blood sugar (hypoglycaemia) → Hunger/irritability → (back to Eating refined carbohydrates)

Just when you thought it couldn't get worse, it does! Insulin has many essential functions in maintaining life, but it has one very bad action for the dieter: *it causes excess carbohydrate to be stored as fat.* In other words, it actually stimulates the deposit of fat around our bodies.

Let us go over this again, just to be certain that you fully understand the mechanism of fat storage in the body, because by shutting down this mechanism, you reverse the process: instead of making fat, you burn fat.

- When you are hungry, you eat carbohydrates, which provide a rapid source of energy.
- This stimulates the production of insulin by the body, which quickly lowers the blood sugar, making you feel weak and irritable, so you eat more carbohydrates to make you feel better, which it does – but only briefly.
- Insulin then stimulates the deposit of excess carbohydrate as fat, especially around the waist and hips. Even worse, it actually prevents body fat from being used to provide energy, so you can never break down body fat if insulin levels are elevated.

Breaking the cycle

How can you put an end to this vicious circle? If you don't eat, you become weaker and weaker (and more irritable), as you all know. The answer is simple:

Reduce the insulin!

If you decrease the amount of insulin your body releases, your blood glucose levels won't plummet so dramatically, so you won't become weak and irritable, and you won't feel the need to eat more carbohydrate for energy. Ultimately, therefore, you won't deposit the fat on your waist and hips.

Even better, if you lower your insulin levels, the body's mechanisms are actually directed to burn body fat preferentially. In other words, you have switched on the body's automatic fat-burning mechanism. Just one small problem. How exactly do you achieve this minor miracle of lowering the insulin level, and therefore converting to 'fat-burning' mode (instead of the usual 'fat-deposit' mode)? Once again, the answer is very simple:

Reduce your intake of refined carbohydrates

The production of insulin is essentially controlled by carbohydrate intake, not fats or proteins, so if you cut down drastically on refined carbohydrates, your insulin levels reduce naturally, and you start to burn body fat. It really is that easy.

All of a sudden, you can now clearly see why previous diets have failed. Almost all diets instruct you to *increase* your daily intake of carbohydrates, usually as cereals, grains, pasta, rice and pulses (peas and beans). Even if you reduce your calorie intake to below the level you need each day, unless you switch off the insulin (and convert to the mode of burning body fat) there is always the tendency to deposit some of the food as more fat. That is what insulin does, and insulin is stimulated by carbohydrates. So you weren't a failure after all, it just was not medically possible to lose weight safely on some of the diets you followed. The system for burning fat was switched off.

Reduce carbohydrate – not calories – to lose weight

Identical calorie intake

Low carbohydrate diet   High carbohydrate diet

Weight loss   Weight gain

Of course, we certainly do not want to switch off our insulin completely; we need insulin, but our bodies do not need, and were never designed to cope with, large quantities of refined carbohydrates, such as the immense loads of refined sugars and starches in the pre-packaged foods that form the basis of the modern Western diet. If we cut out the foods that our bodies cannot safely tolerate, insulin production returns to its normal level, we burn any excess fat and return to our normal shape. You don't see fat animals in nature, because animals don't eat our diet.

There is one other very important point that is going to become quite obvious in a moment. If you switch on your automatic fat-burning mechanism by cutting out refined carbohydrates and sugars, what else do you have to restrict in the diet? NOTHING! Yes, that's right, your eyes are not deceiving you: there are absolutely no other restrictions in the diet. You can eat virtually as much as you like of any other foods, and you will still lose fat. This is hard to believe, but true. For the first time, you are using the body's own established mechanisms to lose fat. So you are *not* going to be hungry, or irritable, or spend all of your time counting calories, and as you will be eating a diet high in protein, vitamins and minerals, your body will be receiving healthy nutrition while losing fat.

Chapter 3 — The principles of the New High Protein Diet

This diet is the most effective way of losing body fat. Remember, if we go on a starvation diet (which is all that many so-called diets are), we lose *weight* but not much *fat*. In starvation mode, we use up our energy stores of carbohydrate first (in the form of a substance called glycogen). However, the body can store only a little glycogen, and this is used up within two days. Then we start breaking down fat and protein. But we can't afford to lose body proteins: our muscle mass decreases, we become noticeably weaker, and our immunity is compromised because the lack of protective immunoglobulin proteins means we are subject to an increased risk of infection. Not good!

Sure, we look slimmer (because our body shape *under* the fat layer is smaller), and we certainly weigh less (because muscle is much heavier than fat), but we are weaker and becoming unhealthy. There is no point in dieting if it's going to make us ill. And, of course, because we need our muscles, when we even slightly stray from the diet, our bodies immediately rebuild muscle and we regain all of the 'lost' weight very quickly. Yet another diet fails – because it was never going to work in the first place. And we have succeeded in making ourselves considerably less healthy in the process. Not only have we gone through a period of reduced immunity and a lack of proteins, minerals, vitamins, antioxidants and other essential nutrients, there is evidence that so-called 'yo-yo' dieting of this nature is detrimental to health in the longer term.

Unlike calorie-control diets, the New High Protein Diet will work, and it is very easy to implement

Quite simply, we are going to virtually eliminate all refined carbohydrates and sugars (which are also carbohydrates), leaving us with a low-carbohydrate, high-protein diet. Of course, you may have heard of (and probably tried) high-protein diets before, and they all failed *because the carbohydrates were not restricted.* Remember, unless you switch off the mechanism to make fat, and switch on the mechanism to burn fat, it is very difficult to lose body fat. On this diet, you will be cutting out virtually all refined carbohydrates (which your body does not need) so that body fat is burned preferentially, to provide energy.

What are refined carbohydrates?

Sugar, starch, white flour, cakes, bread, pasta and rice are the usual culprits. These foods have very little nutritional value and, what's more, can cause medical and fat problems. Of course, there are forms of these carbohydrates – such as wholemeal rice, wholemeal bread and wholemeal pasta – that do have nutritional benefits and which you can reintroduce later, but in the initial stage of the diet, you have to reduce *all* carbohydrates, to switch on the fat-burning mechanism.

Everything containing refined carbohydrates is excluded

A list of foods containing refined carbohydrates can be found on pages 293–7 but you should definitely cut out all pasta, rice, cakes and biscuits, and stick to a maximum of one slice of bread per day. Your body will rapidly adjust to a healthy, high-protein, low-carbohydrate diet, and will burn body fat. The bottom line is that you don't need refined carbohydrates and processed sugars. These foods provide energy (which you can easily obtain from better sources) and no other form of essential nutrition – and when you eat more than the energy you can use immediately, the rest is stored as fat.

One point to be aware of is that refined carbohydrates can appear in many unexpected sources. You probably know that bread, cakes, pastries, biscuits, pies, pizzas, potato crisps and fried potato chips all contain refined carbohydrates, but pasta, rice, most breakfast cereals, most tinned foods, many pre-packaged foods, tinned vegetables, tinned soups, and prepared sauces do as well . . . In fact, the list goes on and on. Virtually all 'fast foods' contain very high proportions of refined carbohydrates – as well as hydrogenated fats – and if your diet is high in refined carbohydrates and hydrogenated fats, you will definitely put on weight.

If you're worried that by cutting out refined carbohydrates you'll have virtually no foods left to choose from, fear not. In fact, high-protein and nutritious foods such as meat, poultry, fish, shellfish and eggs are all open to you, along with vegetables, cheese, spices and herbs, from which you can easily produce delicious, healthy and quick meals. You'll be relieved to hear that you don't have to live on a diet of lettuce and tomato (nutritious as they are, they are rather limited in taste on their own). On the contrary, you will be eating virtually *limitless* quantities of very tasty food, complemented by delicious sauces and dressings: in other words, real food! To demonstrate just how easily this can be achieved, a comprehensive list of recipes is included in Part II of the book, all of which can easily be incorporated into your busy lifestyle. In short, you'll eat well and still lose fat.

What about fats in your diet? I've advised you to cut out refined carbohydrates and eat a high-protein diet, but what about the amount of fat you consume? This is going to seem a strange thing to say, and it's against all of the dietary advice you've been given in the past, but if you follow the principles of this diet carefully, *you don't need worry about how much fat you're consuming.* No, I have not gone mad, and I'm certainly not advocating a high-fat diet, but most of the 'bad' fats are actually integrated into the sugary, starchy foods you have already excluded, and you will naturally avoid them when you stop eating these foods. So by excluding the refined carbohydrates, you have excluded the 'bad' fats from your diet at a single stroke.

Not all fats are bad

Some fats are actually essential for life. We need fats to make part of the outer walls around cells in the body (of which there are trillions), to produce the sheaths of nerve cells, and to make hormones that are essential for life. In addition, certain essential vitamins are fat-soluble, which means that you need fat to absorb them. I'm not, of course, suggesting that you will be healthier on a diet of burgers and French fries (which you have just excluded from your diet anyway), but the flip side of the coin is that you also will not be healthy without essential fats in your diet. The secret is knowing which are the essential fats (which incidentally have the most taste) and which are the ones to avoid. Most 'fast' foods are cooked in 'trans' fats, which are definitely not good for your health.

The old story that if you eat fat you will get fat is only true if you *also* eat carbohydrates. If you don't eat carbohydrates, you will switch off the fat-making process to a large extent, and fats in the diet do not switch it on. So you can eat more fats of the correct type in these circumstances, without weight gain, and actually mobilise your own excess body fat in the process.

Fats in our diet, apart from being essential for many body functions, also play an important role in digestion. They *slow* the absorption process in the intestine, preventing the highs and lows of blood sugar levels produced by carbohydrates and insulin, so we feel more stable and have less acute mood swings. Fats in the diet make us feel satisfied after a meal, preventing the hunger pangs that are experienced within an hour or two of a carbohydrate-based meal. And finally, the body tells us when to stop eating 'pure' fats (unlike the fats combined with sugars in, for example, cakes and chocolate, which can be quite addictive). In fact, we only overindulge in fats when they are combined with sugars or starches (such as in potato chips). I have never heard of a case of overeating associated purely with butter, cheese, avocados, fresh nuts, eggs, or animal or fish products. On the contrary, many natural oils are healthy. An excellent example is fish oils, which have been clearly proven to be very good for us – and no one ever heard of a fat fish! Personally, I do not particularly like the taste of excess animal fat, so I would still recommend lean meat; the amount of saturated fat in a lean cut of meat is certainly not excessive.

So you can clearly see that if you cut out refined carbohydrates from your diet, you simultaneously exclude most of the 'bad' fats, lose body fat, feel better, look better, and actually get significantly healthier – without being hungry or tired. What could be easier?

A two-step programme

What? No bread or pasta or cakes or rice, for ever! No more chips, or burgers, or steak pies? It's not worth living; I can hear the storm of protest from some of you already. No, don't worry. You don't have to forsake all of these culinary delights for ever. Remember, this is a fat reduction diet. You have to get rid of the excess fat that you have accumulated over the years, so obviously you have to avoid fattening foods at the moment, but you can eat them at a later stage *in moderation*. Your first goal is to remove the causes of fat accumulation in the first place, but once you have lost your excess fat (and it will go faster than you expect on this diet) then you can include some of these desirable (if unhealthy) foods, but in much smaller proportions than before. I'm not suggesting that you never again eat cake or ice cream – just not during the diet!

In essence, this means that there are two stages to the diet: a weight-loss stage and a weight-maintenance stage. In the first stage (weight loss), you have to keep strictly to the 40–60 gram daily limit for carbohydrates to lose weight quickly. When you have reached your target size, or when the weight loss has stopped (which is your body telling you that this is the correct weight for you and you won't lose any more weight safely), you can increase your carbohydrate intake again, in moderation (the weight maintenance stage). Your body will quickly tell you if you're eating too much carbohydrate, because you'll gain weight. The amount of carbohydrate really is different for everyone, but you'll almost certainly be able to eat more than 60 grams per day without weight gain.

In effect, this simply means that after you have lost weight, providing you eat refined carbohydrates in moderation, you will not gain weight as fat. But I can assure you that after you have re-programmed your body on this healthy, satisfying diet, you will no longer be addicted to sugar and starchy foods – because that is what this is, a mild form of addiction which your body has developed in response to fluctuating sugar levels and the associated fluctuating insulin levels.

After only a few days on this diet, you will find that you are not as hungry as before, not only because you are eating sufficient amounts to stave off hunger, but also because you have literally re-programmed your body to a more normal desire for food. This is a natural consequence of a high-protein, low-carbohydrate diet. In many cases, individuals find that they still enjoy carbohydrates after the diet, but they no longer need them in such large quantities. The diet is effective in the longer term because your eating patterns are re-set. You no longer have to think about what you must not eat; the intense desire is no longer there, so it's easy to resist. Many people find they have simply lost the taste for the 'bad' foods, which makes keeping slim so much easier.

It is much easier to prevent the fat from re-accumulating after this diet, because you have actually lost most of your excess fat in the first place. As you now appreciate, calorie-control seldom works in actually losing fat, because the mechanism for fat storage has not been switched off. So you can return to some of your old ways, and if you only eat the 'bad' foods in moderation, you probably won't put on weight.

A new sense of well-being

You will have noticed that I continually use the term 'fat' instead of 'weight'. There are two reasons for this: firstly, the weight you are losing is actually fat on this diet, unlike the loss of weight as body protein on other diets; and secondly, the word 'fat' is very emotive. It embodies the feeling of dislike (almost disgust) that the dieter feels towards this excess tissue. Instead of disguising this unpleasant feeling with inaccurate terms like 'weight loss', I believe that the most important step is to accept the problem at face value – physically, psychologically and emotionally. There are few more emotive subjects in Western society than body fat.

On this diet, you will re-educate your body to accept and enjoy healthier food, which actually tastes better, because you will be shown how easy it is and how good you feel. And this second point is very important: you *will* feel better. Not just because you have succeeded in losing fat and you look much better, but also because you will be – and feel – healthier. You will be able to return to a much less restricted diet after you have lost the fat you wanted to lose, because the fat has gone, whereas on previous diets the fat was still there, merely disguised by the slimming effects of loss of muscle and body protein.

But to rid yourself of excess body fat is not enough. My aim is to ensure that you are much healthier, and that is why the diet is divided into two stages:

- In the early stage – excess weight-loss phase – you concentrate on getting rid of the fat. Carbohydrates *must* be severely restricted in this phase for effective and rapid weight loss.
- In the later stage – the weight-maintenance phase – when you are satisfied with your weight, you are allowed a much more liberal diet, because it's much more difficult to gain weight (as fat) when you exclude most of the refined carbohydrates. This means that you can eat far more foods than you ever thought possible, remain healthy, and not deposit additional adipose tissue (medicalspeak for fat).

Losing weight safely

It is very important that you do not reduce in size too quickly. I know everyone wants to lose the fat as quickly as possible – and this diet will work quite rapidly – but you shouldn't try to accelerate the effect of the diet by reducing the amounts you eat. This is a common mistake among dieters, and will lead to inevitable failure. This diet will reduce weight – as fat – *at the most efficient rate for your body*. It is much faster than other diets, and it results in definite loss of fat (and not protein) if followed correctly. But if you tamper with the rules, it won't work, because it depends entirely upon switching off the fat-storage mechanisms in the body. For example, if you add in one or two cakes, or biscuits, or bars of chocolate, this diet will fail because your carbohydrate intake will be too high. It is also important that you do not reduce your weight too rapidly because:

- It is not healthy, and can make you very sick, with reduced immunity from infection. This high-protein diet will ensure that does not happen.

- If you lose weight too quickly, your skin doesn't have enough time to adapt to the new, smaller you, and you will be left with unsightly folds of excess skin.

How many times have you read of dieters requiring surgery after severe dieting? It is obviously ridiculous to require surgery – and have surgical scars and possible post-operative complications – as a result of a diet that was intended to make you look more attractive! If you reduce in size at a regular pace – usually 1–1.5 kilos per week initially – you will achieve a much better final cosmetic appearance, which is the aim of the diet. By restricting refined carbohydrates, you will lose weight steadily *and at the fastest rate your body can withstand while still remaining healthy*. More importantly, you will continue to lose weight at a rate of about 1 kilo per week until you approach the 'normal' weight for your height and shape, which is genetically pre-programmed in all of us from birth. At this point, weight loss will slow down – in other words, your genes determine your normal shape, as long as you supply your body with the necessary nutrition in the correct proportions. The mechanism is already in place: you just have to provide the building blocks and your genes will do the rest.

Chapter 4 The golden rules for a successful diet

Now that you understand the basis of this new system of eating (and therefore dieting), you can begin the process of removing excess fat for ever. The beauty of this system is that your body's hormones do the work for you. In other words, your body will automatically reduce your weight to the level that is right for you, at the safest healthy rate for the human body, then automatically stop. You are not artificially manipulating your body (as on other diets), you are simply allowing your body's hormones to remove excess body fat medically. Obviously, you must have a realistic body image – waif-like proportions are not normal – but neither is the fat created by a modern diet of refined carbohydrates. You will lose weight easily by simply following the rules. Conversely, you won't lose too much weight on this diet. You are consuming high-quality protein and essential fats, vitamins and minerals, and when you reach your correct body weight, your hormones simply switch off the weight loss process; it seems too good to be true but it isn't. You provide the correct ingredients, as healthy food, and nature does the rest.

However, before commencing any diet you should discuss the matter with your GP, to ensure that there are no medical problems which make dieting unsafe for you. There are obvious situations, like pregnancy, where dieting is definitely contraindicated, but there are also many other conditions in which dieting may not be safe, and which may not be obvious to you. So always obtain your doctor's advice before dieting – or exercising.

As mentioned in a previous chapter, the diet consists of two parts: a weight-loss phase and a weight-maintenance phase. In the weight-loss phase, you must restrict carbohydrates to less than 60 grams per day (and preferably less than 40 grams per day) to lose weight. When you are satisfied with your size (and try to base your decision on *size* not *weight),* or when the weight loss stops (which is your body's way of saying that this is your correct size), go on to the weight-maintenance phase of the diet. I have emphasised *size* rather than *weight* because you are losing fat on this diet (which, of course, is exactly what you want), but fat is much lighter than protein, so you will reduce in *size* more than you reduce in *weight.* In fact, weight is a dreadful way of measuring the success of a diet, because, generally, the more weight you lose, the more body protein you lose, which is very dangerous.

As this system is really a way of life rather than a diet, you will find by the weight maintenance stage that you no longer crave refined carbohydrates, and it should be reasonably easy to keep your weight stable, even though you are consuming more (but not too much more) than 60 grams of carbohydrate per day. If you find your weight creeping back up, cut down the carbohydrates and it will soon reduce.

How to cut down on carbohydrates

As you will have appreciated by now, this medically based diet works by switching on the fat-burning mechanism we each have as an intrinsic part of our body chemistry. If you switch off the fat-storage mechanism, and switch on the fat-burning mechanism, you will lose fat. This depends entirely upon severely restricting your carbohydrate intake, especially in the early stages of the diet, because it is primarily carbohydrates (not fat or proteins) that stimulate insulin production – the hormone that promotes fat storage. So there is no possibility of 'cheating', even a little, on this diet. If you include the occasional cake or chocolate or pasta, the diet will not work.

So, the number one rule of the diet is as follows:

Eat no more than 40–60 grams of carbohydrate a day

Ideally you should try to keep below 40 grams of carbohydrate per day, and certainly below 60 grams. A single slice of bread alone is 17 grams of carbohydrate, so you can see that the carbohydrate limit is very strict. Of course, no one is perfect and you are bound to break the rules occasionally, but you *must* try to keep to less than an absolute maximum of 60 grams of carbohydrate per day. If you exceed this level, the insulin response is almost certainly going to be activated, and suddenly all of the unlimited amounts of high-protein foods in your diet will be deposited as fat, and the fat-burning mechanism is switched off.

In practice, this means no breakfast cereals, milk (though cheese is allowed), cakes, biscuits, pies, potato crisps, potato chips, or most refined pre-packaged foods – and virtually no bread. It also means no refined sugar of any nature. And definitely no potatoes, pasta or rice.

These foods are very high in carbohydrate content, and must be avoided completely in the weight-loss stage of the diet. Later, you can re-introduce limited amounts of wholemeal bread, wholemeal pasta and wholemeal rice, which are rich in vitamins (such as thiamin) and fibre. Wholemeal products slow the digestive process, helping to prevent the massive fluctuations in blood sugar levels which are characteristic of the absorption of foods made from white, refined flour. Potatoes have a high starch component, and although they are an excellent source of nutrition, they must be avoided initially to reduce the insulin response and promote fat loss.

But to keep to the 40-gram limit, you also have to be wary of some other foods, as follows:

Restrict fruit in the weight-loss stage of the diet

I dislike this rule, but unfortunately it is necessary at first. All fruit is good for you. It is full of vitamins, minerals and fibre, and has a very high antioxidant capacity. Unfortunately for the dieter, many fruits also have a high sugar content. Now, these sugars are *natural* rather than *refined*, and are therefore much better for you than those found in cakes and sweets, but the insulin response cannot differentiate between one type of sugar and another, so you do have to limit severely the amount of fruit you eat in the weight-loss stage of the diet. If possible, omit fruit entirely from your diet, apart from an orange per day to maintain safe vitamin C levels. Of course, if you take a diet supplement tablet which contains your daily requirement of vitamin C, you could replace the orange with another piece of fruit, such as an apple or a peach. Check the table on page 294 to find out the carbohydrate content of various fruits. In general, most pieces of fruit contain 10–15 grams of carbohydrate each, so be careful. Bananas, however, are definitely out. As soon as you proceed to the weight-maintenance stage of the diet, re-introduce fruit at the earliest possible opportunity.

Vitamin C is essential for good health and has many important actions, not least its wonderful antioxidant properties. It is one of the few nutrients that we cannot obtain from animal foods (apart from liver). Although many vegetables are excellent sources of the vitamin, citrus fruits are the simplest way of preventing deficiency; a single orange provides your daily requirement of vitamin C – hence the one-orange-a-day allowance during the weight-loss phase of this diet. You will notice that many of the suggested recipes incorporate fresh lemon or lime juice, both for flavour and nutrition. However, even a single orange contains about 15 grams of carbohydrate (about the same as one slice of bread), and you have to keep your daily carbohydrate intake to less than 40 grams per day, if possible, to continue the fat-burning mechanism. So if you can replace the orange (or lemon) with a vitamin C supplement in tablet form, you will significantly reduce your daily carbohydrate intake.

No fruit juices

Fruit juices are high in sugar content (even the 'unsweetened' variety) and are totally excluded from this diet. This includes *all* fruit juices, commercial and freshly squeezed; they may have different sugar contents, but they all have too much sugar for a low-carbohydrate diet. You will obtain all the vitamins, minerals and antioxidants you need from other components of this diet.

Cut out virtually all milk – even skimmed milk

This restriction is so important that it is worth emphasising, as it is one of the commonest reasons for the failure of a low-carbohydrate diet; the sugar in milk is often forgotten. All milk, even low-fat skimmed varieties, has a high carbohydrate content (as lactose). So if you drink milk, you will exceed the acceptable carbohydrate intake. You can allow yourself perhaps a very little milk in tea, but no more.

The main value of milk is as a source of calcium and vitamins, which are easily provided by the cheese and other constituents in your diet. Cheese and cream are unrestricted because they are virtually carbohydrate-free, so they don't upset the diet. In effect, no carbohydrate, no problem.

No pulses or grains in the weight-loss stage of the diet

Once again, I dislike this restriction, because pulses and whole grains are rich in proteins, vitamins and minerals. Unfortunately, however, they also have a high carbohydrate content, so you'll need to cut them out to begin with. But as soon as the weight-loss phase of the diet is over, you can start cooking with them again.

Stick to low-calorie soft drinks

This particularly refers to carbonated fizzy drinks. This is not because regular soft drinks are high in calories but because they have a high sugar – and therefore a high carbohydrate – content. If you would like a soft drink, use the low-calorie equivalent to prevent sugar from creating an insulin response. But remember, some diet carbonated drinks contain caffeine, which also stimulates the insulin response, so drink them in moderation. Better still, drink water.

Cut out beer

Alcohol is not prohibited on this diet, but beer is definitely out. Beer has a relatively high sugar content (maltose), and will seriously compromise the diet. Wine and spirits have a much lower carbohydrate content (spirits have virtually none), so they can be tolerated in the diet. I know it seems strange, because alcohol is well known to contain lots of calories, but the calorie content is not important in itself on a low-carbohydrate diet. If the carbohydrate content is restricted, the insulin response will be blunted, and the calories in alcohol will not be deposited as fat.

I certainly do not intend to promote alcohol consumption, but I have to tell you the facts as they are, and on this basis a moderate amount of alcohol (as wine or spirits) will not cause weight gain on this diet. In fact, there is significant evidence to suggest that a glass of red wine per day is actually beneficial in preventing long-term heart disease; the protective effect is thought to result from the antioxidants in the red wine. And a 120ml glass of red wine contains less than 1 gram of carbohydrate. The carbohydrate content of various alcoholic beverages is shown on page 301. A word of warning though:

always check the carbohydrate content of *mixer* drinks, which are usually much higher in carbohydrates than is alcohol alone. Low-calorie mixers are your best choice.

One other point to remember is that alcohol generally increases the appetite and affects self-control, so if you drink too much you may eat more than you need or blow your diet by giving in to a carbohydrate craving. In other words, alcohol is not necessarily bad for either you or your diet – if taken *in moderation*.

Drink tea, not coffee

Try to avoid coffee, or at least reduce your intake considerably, not just because of the effects of caffeine, but because *coffee stimulates insulin production*. In other words, coffee accelerates the effects of carbohydrates by magnifying the insulin response. And insulin promotes fat storage. So stop drinking coffee to help you lose weight – even though coffee, by itself, has no calorie content.

Fortunately, nature has provided us with a perfect substitute – tea. Unlike coffee, tea has no untoward effects on sugar metabolism, and so it does not upset our fat-losing programme. And tea has very high levels of antioxidants. It was always presumed that green tea was healthier than dark tea in this respect, but recent research has shown very little difference between the two types in terms of antioxidant levels. Drink tea – but with either very little milk (preferably none), or with cream, which has no carbohydrate content, rather than milk. Lemon in tea tastes great and is nutritionally excellent.

So those are the foods you need to avoid. But one word of advice: don't exclude carbohydrates completely from your diet. Have the equivalent of a slice of bread per day. There are also complex carbohydrates in the vegetables included in the diet. If you abstain from carbohydrates completely, you will notice a strange taste in your mouth. This is down to substances called ketones, which are the breakdown products of fats, and are a warning that you are reducing the carbohydrates a little too much. If you would rather not have a slice of bread, you can substitute another carbohydrate food for this, examples of which are shown in the table on pages 293–4.

And here's what you can eat . . .

Although carbohydrate foods are out, there are still hundreds of delicious meals for you to enjoy, such as trout with lemon hollandaise sauce, pepper steak, moussaka, beef stroganoff, sweet and sour pork, lamb curry with red pepper, roast beef . . . The potential variations with this diet are literally endless, and I have included lots of ideas and delicious recipes for putting the diet into practice in Part II of the book.

Don't worry, within a very short period you won't miss carbohydrates. Your body will automatically readjust to a healthy diet (which is one with no refined carbohydrates) and the addiction to sugars (because that's what it is) will simply disappear. That is the reason why you have to give up virtually all carbohydrates, because if you cheat then your body doesn't have a chance to readjust.

Have as much protein as you like

There is no restriction on *fresh* beef, pork, lamb, poultry, fish (including shellfish), eggs or cheese (except some of the processed cheeses). I have emphasised that this applies to fresh animal products only, to differentiate from pre-packaged foods, which can contain large quantities of hidden carbohydrates and sugars.

Manufactured foods such as sausages can vary enormously in their carbohydrate content; some contain high proportions of carbohydrates, whereas others (such as Polish kabanas) have virtually no carbohydrate content at all – so you should try to acquire the simple habit of reading the carbohydrate content on the labels. 'Pure' proteins (meat, poultry, fish, shellfish and eggs) have virtually no carbohydrate content, so it's much easier to base your diet on these foods. As well as being the basis of a successful weight-loss diet, they are also full of healthy nutrients and flavour.

This does not mean that you will gorge yourself on protein foods; your metabolism will not allow this. In fact, we only overindulge in carbohydrate foods – or, more specifically, combinations of carbohydrates and fats, which is where the problem arises. We do not overindulge in 'pure' fats; our metabolism tells us when to stop, because fats satisfy hunger. If carbohydrates did the same, there wouldn't be a problem.

Plants, of course, are an excellent source of protein (although usually not 'complete' proteins. The exception is soya (and its derivatives), which is certainly a complete protein.

Don't worry about 'pure' fats

This is the strangest rule of all. You are on a diet, and not restricting fats! Well you *are* actually restricting fats, and particularly the 'bad' fats in your diet, by severely restricting the carbohydrates, because the worst fats in your diet are combined with carbohydrates – which, of course, you have eliminated. Your body automatically adjusts to the new equilibrium, and you will not suddenly gorge on butter, cheese, cream and eggs. Your body knows when to stop, and, just in case this mechanism is faulty, you have switched off the fat-storage hormone so you will excrete any excess fat from your body and not store it as extra fat.

Before you become overly concerned about the fat in your diet (which we have changed from 'bad' fats to 'good' fats), perhaps I should mention that there is a considerable body of medical evidence supporting the hypothesis that simply lowering the amount of cholesterol you consume will not necessarily lower your blood cholesterol level. In other words, eating a low-fat diet does not equate to having a low blood cholesterol level. I know this seems like dietary heresy after all you have been told about how essential it is to adhere strictly to a low-fat diet for your future health, but as a clinician I have to present the facts, and the facts are that many highly respected medical journals have recently published scientific papers that strongly refute the concept of 'low dietary fat equals low cholesterol and better health'. In simple terms, all fats are definitely *not* bad for you.

One final point. In my opinion, eggs get a very bad press from certain dietary 'experts'. This is because egg yolks contain cholesterol. Now, let us remember that we need a certain amount of cholesterol for many essential body functions (hormone production, nervous system functioning – including the brain – and cell membrane formation, to name but a few), so all cholesterol is not bad. Major studies of healthy adults have shown that one egg a day does not increase the risk of heart disease and stroke, and that two eggs a day actually increase the amount of 'good' cholesterol in your blood, which is protective against heart disease. So eggs are not bad for us. And just think of all of the nutrition in an egg; it is a source of many essential amino acids, antioxidants, vitamins and minerals – and the proportion of the various nutrients in an egg are exactly in proportion to our nutritional requirements. How typical of nature to get it right, and of us to get it wrong! I am not suggesting that you overindulge in eggs, but an egg per day is not harmful, and has so many amazing health benefits that it is incredible that eggs have been criticised in the first place.

Feast on fresh vegetables
Fresh vegetables have so much goodness that it is difficult to know where to begin listing the benefits. They provide vitamins

and minerals in abundance, and therefore many of the essential antioxidants we need to protect against disease and infection.

Basically, you can include virtually all vegetables in your diet, apart from those high in starch, such as potatoes, parsnips, corn and pulses (peas, beans and lentils) – see Appendix 2 for a detailed list. The list of vegetables included in the diet far outweighs those excluded.

It is essential that you don't ruin the nutrition contained in vegetables by inappropriate cooking. Vitamins and minerals are lost from vegetables when they are chopped up too early, so prepare them just before you intend to cook them. Of course, this isn't always practical, in which case a sealed packet of pre-chopped fresh vegetables (which retain a significant amount of goodness) is an acceptable substitute. Nutrients also leach out when you boil vegetables in water, so try to steam them, cook them in just a small amount of water, or, better still, use a wok, as this method of cooking retains a lot of the inherent goodness in foods (for more on wok cooking, sees pages 54–5).

So there you have the rules of the diet. What could be simpler? If you are in any doubt as to which foods you can eat and which are best avoided, you will find several charts in the book. A list of 'forbidden' foods is shown on pages 42–3, and these should be avoided at all times during the weight-loss stage of the diet. In the maintenance stage, you can have some of the 'forbidden foods', in moderation, but remember, your body will have readjusted and you will no longer have carbohydrate cravings. The list is not all-inclusive, as sugars and other carbohydrates can be 'hidden', so read the label on any pre-packaged or processed food to check the carbohydrate content.

To help you stick to the 40-gram carbohydrate limit, lists of the typical carbohydrate content of common foods are shown on pages 293–7; the first list details foods with a low carbohydrate content which can be included in the diet, and the second details those with a high carbohydrate content which should be excluded. For example, if you have a 100-gram slice of chocolate cake (carbohydrate content 55 grams) or a 100-gram bar of milk chocolate (carbohydrate content 61 grams), you have already exceeded your carbohydrate allowance for the day. But if you have an apple (13 grams carbohydrate), a peach (9 grams carbohydrate) or a shortbread biscuit (11 grams carbohydrate), you'll be within the allowance. The recipes in Part II of the book will help you to create delicious meals within the daily 40-gram carbohydrate limit; you'll see that the carbohydrate content of each dish is indicated at the end of each recipe.

It's actually easier to *stop* eating refined carbohydrates completely (as you lose the taste for them) than to cut down your carbohydrate intake, but if you can't stop, use the tables on pages 293–300 for guidance in keeping your daily intake below 40 grams. If you follow the general guidelines of the diet, you won't have to count carbohydrate content at all, and I can assure you that you will be receiving all the necessary ingredients for healthy nutrition, too. Indeed, you will be eating highly nutritious natural food, and be slimming at the fastest *safe* rate for your body – the perfect combination for the serious slimmer!

The weight-maintenance phase

There is no 'after the diet', there is only 'after the weight loss'. This is a way of life, not just a new fad diet to lose body fat. If you adhere to the rules, you will lose fat, you will probably be eating a healthier diet than ever before, and you will find you no longer need your sugar fix. As I mentioned earlier, there is no definite carbohydrate limit at this stage of the diet, because everyone has a different tolerance for carbohydrates. You can gradually re-introduce fruit, root vegetables, pulses and milk, and, providing your weight doesn't increase, you're quite safe. Obviously, even the 'forbidden' foods (like cakes and pastries) can be reintroduced *in moderation,* but, as previously mentioned, you'll find that you don't *need* them as you did before, and you'll probably not over-indulge.

So the end of the weight-loss phase is signalled either by your satisfaction that you have lost sufficient weight (and you definitely will lose weight on this diet, unlike others), or when the weight loss stops, which is the body telling you to stop trying to lose weight. Once you are satisfied with your weight and shape (and *please* be realistic about your aims), you can reintroduce certain foods, which you had to restrict during the weight-loss phase because of their carbohydrate content but which are nevertheless excellent sources of nutrition:

- *Fresh fruit.* All fresh fruit is full of vitamins and minerals, and therefore high in antioxidants. Fruit can be re-introduced in moderation (preferably no more than two standard pieces per day) when you are satisfied with your weight.
- *Whole grains.* These foods are high in B vitamins (thiamin, riboflavin and niacin), vitamin A and vitamin E.
- *Full-cream milk and milk products.* Milk is like eggs: it naturally contains all the nutrients you need and in the correct proportions for health. It is well known to be an excellent source of calcium and vitamin D (for strong bones), but it also provides vitamins A, B_2, B_6 and B_{12}.

  Why do I always suggest full-cream milk instead of low-fat milk? Surely low-fat skimmed milk is healthier, with the same calcium content but lower fat content? Unfortunately, the mechanics of the body are not that simple; it *needs* fat to absorb both calcium and vitamin D, so if you drink low-fat milk, you actually absorb less than 10 per cent of the calcium, which rather tends to defeat the purpose of drinking milk! Use full-cream milk and you *will* absorb the necessary calcium and vitamin D.

- *Pulses.* Beans, peas and lentils are excellent sources of proteins. Although they are not 'complete' proteins (like animal proteins) they are easily elevated to 'complete' status by combining them with either whole grains or milk.

All of the nutrition contained in these temporarily excluded food groups is provided by alternative foods in the diet, so you will not be missing any of the necessary proteins, vitamins and minerals during the weight-loss stage of the diet. Fruit, milk, whole grains and pulses are very good sources of nutrition which are only being restricted for a short time to allow you to lose your unwanted body fat.

In fact, the only foods that you should severely restrict for ever are those consisting mainly of refined carbohydrates, our old 'friends' the cakes, pies, pastries, commercial pizza (you can make a healthy one at home), crisps, chips (once again, you can make oven-cooked chipped potatoes at home) and most commercial 'fast' foods – but home-made burgers can be among the most nutritious of foods. And the word is *restrict* not *omit*: you can have some foods with refined carbohydrates in your daily diet after you have lost weight – just reduce them to a low level of consumption and you should be fine. Your body will soon tell you if you're eating too much, because you'll put on weight.

What happens if you break your diet occasionally?

Unfortunately, this diet is not as forgiving as some others. In a calorie-control diet, you can eat some chocolate cake and make up for the extra calories by eating very little for the rest of the day – but low-calorie diets mess up the body's chemical balance and don't work.

In the low-carbohydrate diet, if you consume more than 60 grams of carbohydrate per day, your body will respond by depositing the excess calories as fat. So you can't have many lapses, or it simply won't work. A biscuit here and a pastry there and it will all go to fat. Of course, nobody's perfect (certainly not me!), and no one can rigidly adhere to all the rules all the time. The occasional lapse with a sandwich or a piece of fruit will merely cause the diet to fail on that day only, but really this diet is so liberal that lapses will be infrequent. So don't panic if you break your diet occasionally, it's only human. By satisfying your natural hunger in a natural way, for the first time you have a diet that is working *with* you, not *against* you. Remember, within a few days of commencing the diet your body will automatically readjust, and you will no longer need sugars; the addiction will disappear. Your body will be on automatic pilot! And you will not be hungry during the early phase of the diet, the most difficult period in most diets.

And now to the good part!

After a few weeks on the diet, your body automatically adjusts to the new insulin levels. This means that you will almost certainly be able to eat more than 60 grams of carbohydrate per day after the weight-loss phase of the diet *and still not gain weight*. Obviously you can't eat too much or your weight will increase, but you will be able to 'mini-binge' safely on occasions.

This diet works – and it lasts!

1. Weight-loss phase

Foods excluded from the diet

You'll need to cut out most carbohydrates, to ensure a daily carbohydrate intake of less than 40 grams per day. To avoid the hassle of carbohydrate-counting, which is almost as bad as calorie-counting, this essentially involves excluding the following foods:

- Bread – a maximum of 1 slice (preferably wholemeal) per day
- Pasta
- Rice
- Flour
- Potatoes and certain other starchy vegetables (see page 295)
- Refined sugar of any nature, especially cakes, biscuits, pastries, pies and processed or pre-packaged foods with 'hidden' sugars or carbohydrate content. Read the labels on food to determine how much sugar or carbo-hydrate is in it. Remember, most 'low-fat' foods are high in carbohydrates, so they are not good in this diet
- Breakfast cereals
- Milk (you can have a *very* little in tea, if necessary, but be careful not to ruin your diet with too much). Substitute cream or lemon if possible
- Coffee (if possible). If you can't exclude coffee, drink only decaffeinated coffee. Caffeine stimulates insulin production *without* sugar, so it is definitely not good for this diet
- Beer – far too high in sugar
- Fruits (except an orange or lemon per day) and in the first stage of the diet only. Fruit is re-introduced as

quickly as possible when weight loss is proceeding at a satisfactory pace
- Fruit juice – commercial or freshly squeezed
- Dried fruit
- Pulses (peas, beans, lentils) or grains, in the first stage of the diet. You can re-introduce these in the weight-maintenance phase, when you are satisfied with your weight

Foods included in the diet without restriction on quantity

- All fresh protein from an animal source: beef, poultry, pork, lamb, offal (such as liver), fish and shellfish Tinned tuna, sardines and salmon are also unrestricted
- 'Pure' fats, such as butter, cream, olive oil (especially extra-virgin olive oil), fish oils, nut oils and mayonnaise (without added sugar)
- Fresh vegetables, except those high in starch, such as potatoes. You will find a list of vegetables you can eat at any stage of the diet on pages 299–300, and a list of vegetables you should restrict during the weight-loss phase (primarily root vegetables) on page 300
- Onions, which deserve a special mention, for their high vitamin and mineral content, and excellent antioxidant capacity
- Herbs, especially garlic and ginger
- Spices
- Low-calorie soft drinks (except those restricted by their phenylalanine or caffeine content)
- Tea – an excellent source of protective antioxidants
- Artificial sweeteners – providing they do not incorporate carbohydrates (most don't)

Foods included with some restriction

- Eggs: maximum 5 per week
- Cheese: 50 grams per day
- Yoghurt: natural or Greek yoghurt only, maximum 3 servings per week
- Red/dry white wine: maximum 2 glasses per day, or alcoholic spirits (whisky, gin, brandy): 1 measure per day
- Nuts: 50 grams Brazil nuts, almonds, hazelnuts. Nuts definitely to be excluded are cashew nuts, peanuts and pistachios in the early days of the diet

2. Weight-maintenance phase

Having just told you to cut out all pasta, rice, potatoes and fruits, we are now going to reintroduce these in the weight-maintenance phase. How can this be? Why won't you immediately gain the weight that you have just lost?

Simply because fat is controlled by the hormone insulin, and in the weight-loss phase you have reduced your insulin levels and therefore reintroducing some refined carbohydrate at this stage will not cause weight gain. Remember, this is a *medical diet*, not a fad diet. Of course, if you go wild and binge excessively on bread, pasta, rice and all the other baddies, you certainly will put on weight. But you won't feel the need to have all of these foods in excess, because it was the insulin level that was driving your addiction to these foods and that has now reduced. Now you won't feel like eating as much as before and you will not be so addicted. It is as simple as that. The foods that you can return to your diet in moderation include:

- Bread (up to 30 grams per day)
- Pasta
- Rice (especially arborio rice which is very low GI)

- Fruit (up to 3 pieces per day, which can include a bowl of berries)
- Pulses (especially chick peas which are very healthy)

When you reintroduce these higher-carbohydrate foods in the weight-maintenance phase, you have to count the carbohydrate levels carefully. These are given in Appendix I and II and at the end of each recipe.

Chapter **5** The diet in practice

The beauty of this diet is that you don't have to count calories or settle for small portions. It is also a much easier way of losing weight than standard diets: you eat as much as you like of some foods, restrict carbohydrates, and you lose fat without really trying!

But it will involve a change in the way you think about food. For example, most of us are conditioned to consider carbohydrates as our primary 'fast' food, from cereals and toast with marmalade for breakfast, to pastries or biscuits at mid-morning, sandwiches or fried food at lunchtime, and pasta, rice or potatoes as a standard addition to the evening meal.

The typical carbohydrate-based diet

Breakfast	Mid-morning snack	Lunch	Dinner
cereal	pastries	sandwiches	pasta
toast	biscuits	pasta	pizza
croissants		*take-away*:	curry
marmalade		pies	fish and chips
		Chinese	meat and
		Indian	potatoes
		burgers	*take-away*:
		pizza	(same as lunch)
		fish and chips	

These carbohydrates are self-serving: the more you eat, the more they stimulate insulin which rapidly lowers your blood sugar levels; this in turn makes you crave yet more sugar, which is then deposited as fat. So you need to stop thinking of carbohydrates as the 'main event' of your meals, and base your diet instead on meat, fish, poultry and vegetables. Bread, rice, pasta and potatoes are merely the 'support act'; they provide bulk to your diet – and more energy than you require, which is stored as excess fat. You don't need them, and should therefore exclude them from your diet – at least while you are in the process of losing fat.

Have a substantial breakfast

How many times have you heard that breakfast is the most important meal of the day? This is true, but it's also true that you have to eat the right kind of breakfast, especially if you are trying to lose fat. There is no point filling up on carbohydrates at breakfast – bread, jam, marmalade, cereal, milk and sugar – because they only stimulate an insulin response, your blood sugar drops within 1–2 hours, you become hungry and slightly irritable, and eat more carbohydrates (such as biscuits, pastries or cakes) to compensate. And thus the vicious circle continues.

So when you are actively losing weight, you should stick to an absolute maximum of one slice of bread (or equivalent) per day, and avoid all cereal, grains and sweet food (except fruit, and even that has to be severely restricted during the weight-loss phase) for breakfast. In addition, try to cut out virtually all milk, as it is relatively high in sugar; a little milk in tea or coffee is all that is allowed, and even that should be replaced by cream if possible.

Don't worry, you won't starve without bread and cereals for breakfast; in fact, you won't even be hungry. These will be replaced by eggs (fried, boiled, poached, omelette, scrambled), bacon, gammon, cheese, mayonnaise, mushrooms, chicken, ham, fish (especially smoked) . . . The possibilities are endless! You'll find dozens of mouth-watering breakfast recipes in Part II.

The other reason that you should eat a substantial breakfast low in carbohydrate but with some fat content is because fats satisfy your hunger and slow the absorption of food from the intestines. In other words, you will be satisfied after the meal and won't feel hungry for hours – which is exactly what you are trying to achieve.

The only problem is time. Most of us are in too much of a rush to prepare breakfast first thing in the morning. Or so we are indoctrinated to think! In fact, it takes no longer to cook boiled eggs, or scrambled eggs (very easy in a microwave), poached or fried eggs with toast and either bacon or grilled gammon than it does to eat polystyrene cereal and toast with marmalade. With a breakfast of eggs and bacon (or grilled gammon steak), not only do you start the day with a substantial meal that tastes good, but you also act in the best interests of your health by having a high-protein, low-carbohydrate meal. The protein, vitamins and minerals from the bacon/gammon and eggs cannot be bettered by synthetic foods, and the fat will *naturally* satisfy your hunger for hours by encouraging a slow, steady absorption of food from the bowel, rather than the rapid absorption, and rapid hypoglycaemia, that follows the ingestion of refined carbohydrates. And if you don't like eggs, you can still choose from fish, cold meats, poultry, cheeses . . . Hardly tasteless fare!

Fish may seem a strange thing to eat early in the morning, but kippers or poached fish were popular breakfast dishes until a few decades ago. They taste wonderful, take very little time to cook, and really set you up for the day – they have virtually no carbohydrate content, and contain natural fish oils which slow the absorption of food and are an excellent source of essential fatty acids and antioxidants.

For those who are really pressed for time in the morning, continental ham, sliced meats and poultry, cheese and hard-boiled eggs are marvellous. These need not be expensive. Just two to three slices each of pre-packed ham and cheese with a hard-boiled egg (which cooks itself while you are showering) make an excellent 'fast' breakfast that is also very nutritious and highly 'diet-conscious'.

A wide selection of healthy, nutritious, low-carbohydrate breakfasts is given in Chapter 6.

Light bites and working lunches

It is easy to incorporate lunch into the low-carbohydrate diet. There are several distinct categories of lunch to consider, as different people have different lifestyles: packed lunch, take-away lunch, restaurant lunch and lunch at home. The different approaches to each of these are explained in Chapter 7.

Main meals

More substantial lunches, or dinner, permit an almost infinite array of possibilities, from chicken and pepper frittata to salmon with lemon butter sauce or beef stroganoff. Meals are no longer based on starchy foods, like rice or pasta or potatoes, but rather on nutritious foods such as meat, fish, poultry and vegetables, with delicious sauces to complement the food. An extensive, but by no means comprehensive, list of possible recipes is contained in Part II.

You'll see that there are no desserts in this book. The main reason for this deliberate omission is that you have to break the body's addiction to carbohydrates. If you have dessert, even with low-carbohydrate artificial sweeteners, your body won't be able to readjust, and you won't break the addictive cycle. You have to avoid sweet foods to allow your body to readjust, which it will do in a relatively short period of time.

Safe snacks

Snacking between meals will be less of a problem on this diet than it is on others as your hunger will be naturally satisfied by the foods included in this diet – and it is hunger, not just bad habits, that causes you to snack. In other words, your previous diet failures were *not* your fault: you were simply hungry, and compensated by eating the wrong food. So it really is essential to have a substantial breakfast as this prepares the body for a successful dieting day.

If you must snack, choose judiciously, referring to the lists on pages 293–300 to keep within the 40–60-gram carbohydrate limit. But be careful, it's not worth ruining your diet for the sake of one or two snacks per day. If you are regularly peckish between meals, you probably need to eat more at mealtimes. Providing you stick to the carbohydrate limit, you will not gain weight even if the meals are larger.

There really aren't many safe snacks on a low-carbohydrate diet, because there aren't many snacks that consist of pure protein and fat. By far the best in this regard is nuts, virtually all varieties (except chestnuts and cashew nuts) are low in carbohydrates, have substantial amounts of protein, vitamins and minerals, and are very filling. But I can't emphasise enough that it really is better to eat larger meals to prevent the need for snacking.

Shopping: the secret of successful dieting

All the ingredients for this diet can be planned and purchased on just one shopping trip a week. Your aim is to ensure you always have the following foods to hand:

- *Herbs and spices – fresh and dried.* These not only taste good, but also have a very high concentration of antioxidants, which are essential in the promotion of good health. They do not deposit fat and are easily added to recipes to enhance the taste, so they improve both health and flavour at the same time – simply perfect!

You'll use fresh herbs almost every day, so they won't be wasted. You could also consider growing the herbs yourself, either in your garden or in small pots in the kitchen, for instant availability. Keep a good supply of dried herbs and spices – such as cumin, coriander, turmeric, cinnamon, paprika and chilli – in your store cupboard, too. They can be a little expensive to buy initially, but they last a long time and will enhance countless meals

- *Garlic.* This is one of the most nutritious foods known, with high quantities of vitamins and minerals. It is also an excellent source of antioxidants. So unless you really dislike the taste, try to incorporate garlic in your cooking as often as practically possible. It has been shown to protect against heart disease, cancer and even the ageing process itself through its incredible antioxidant properties
- *Onions*
- *Fresh vegetables*, especially peppers (red, green and yellow, because they have different vitamin concentrations), carrots, broccoli and spring onions
- *Extra-virgin olive oil*
- *Fresh ginger root.* This is a particularly useful herb in many dishes and has marvellous health-giving properties
- *Cheese(s)*, according to taste
- *Soured cream*
- *Mayonnaise*
- *Free-range eggs* – large
- *Fresh beef, poultry, pork or lamb*, according to taste
- *Fresh fish*
- *Tinned tuna* (preferably in brine)
- *Frozen prawns*

- *Oranges and lemons*
- *Tomatoes.* Try to eat these as regularly as possible, as they contain a powerful antioxidant called lycopene, so stock up on both the fresh and tinned varieties. Plum tomatoes have the highest concentration of lycopene, and unusually this health-giving nutrient is actually more prevalent in *cooked* tomatoes than it is in raw ones
- *Black peppercorns*

Other foods that you will need occasionally include:

- *Shellfish*
- *Tomato purée*
- *Dijon mustard*
- *Tomato juice*
- *Nuts* – virtually any kind, according to personal preference: macadamia, almonds, Brazils, walnuts, hazelnuts and occasionally cashew nuts (as these have a much higher carbohydrate content)
- *Limes*

Remember, these ingredients are replacing items you would normally buy, not in addition to your usual shopping bill, so the cost factor is not high. These foods will naturally re-programme your eating habits, so you will begin to require less food without the necessity for either effort or will-power on your part.

Additional recommendations for the diet

The wide variety of foods included without restriction means that this diet is very easy to follow: the guidelines are simple and because you won't feel hungry, you are less likely to deviate from it. You have a very wide latitude in the types of foods that can be included, and Part II provides delicious recipes which are the essence of the diet. Here are a few extra tips to help you adhere to the diet:

Vary your menu as much as possible

You will find the diet easier to stick to if you base your meals on as wide a range of ingredients as possible. Not only are you less likely to get bored (and therefore risk snacking on forbidden carbohydrate foods), but you will also reap greater health benefits. The recipes in Part II of the book have been specially devised to provide as varied a diet as possible. The vegetables have been deliberately selected for their nutritional content: for example, red peppers contain more than 20 times the vitamin C content of lettuce, and more than 15 times the vitamin A content of green peppers. You can follow the standard dietary advice of eating five portions of any fruit or vegetables per day and still not achieve goot nutrition if the fruit and vegetables you choose are not nutritionally balanced. These recipes are specifically designed to ensure excellent nutrition, providing you vary your daily menu. The secret of this diet is that it's not a diet, it's a way of life; if you follow the simple guidelines, you will slim and be nutritionally healthier – with virtually no effort.

Buy a wok

I would strongly advise anyone who wishes to lose fat, or even anyone who just wants to improve his or her health, to buy a wok. Although originating in an ancient era, wok cooking is ideally suited to our modern fast-paced lifestyle, as it allows the rapid cooking of tasty and highly nutritious food. And the variety of meals and combinations of ingredients that can be cooked in this way are almost infinite. For some strange reason, wok cooking seems to be ignored in most slimming recipes, and yet it involves cooking for short periods in small amounts of fat –

and incorporates 'essential' fats which are vital for health. Heat can destroy vitamins, but wok cooking provides intense heat for a relatively short time, 'searing' meat and vegetables and thereby preserving most of the natural goodness in the food.

By cooking in a wok, you finish with a relatively high *volume* but a relatively small *amount* of food, because it has been chopped finely to allow rapid cooking. For example, a carrot, two spring onions, 10–12 florets of broccoli, a red and yellow pepper, a clove of garlic, and two slices of ginger root would be sufficient to provide a very substantial and nutritious vegetable dish for two people. The preparation time is ten minutes, the cooking time is five minutes, and the cost is relatively little. I give this example only to show how quickly, easily and cheaply fresh vegetables can replace pre-packaged 'convenience', foods.

Incidentally, I have no problems with lightly fried food, but I do not ever use deep-fat frying. I don't consider this form of cooking either healthy or necessary in modern society. Whilst sautéing in butter or olive oil is healthy (there really is no medical evidence to the contrary), deep-fat frying can destroy the very nutrition we are aiming to preserve for health.

Get exercising

Regular exercise will complement your diet; not only will it improve your shape and body contour, it will also make you feel much better because regular (simple) exercise improves the blood flow to the tissues of the body, making us look and feel better. You don't need to spend a fortune on a gym membership: simple exercises you can do at home – without expensive equipment – will actually achieve a better result. To this end, I have included a simple programme of isometric exercises on pages 273–291. Isometric means that you can do the exercise in the comfort of your own home (in minutes), and achieve the same result as if you had been to the gym for hours. It needs no equipment and no expertise. It also involves no embarrassment. By investing just 10–12 minutes per day, four days per week, you will improve the muscle tone beneath the disappearing layer of fat, further enhancing the change in body shape which complements the weight-loss programme. If you also walk for 15 minutes three times per week you will improve your cardiovascular health, too. Of course, all exercise programmes *must* be sanctioned by your doctor before you start. For more on the benefits of exercise, and a simple exercise programme, turn to pages 261–71.

Measure shape before weight

I would encourage you to use the changes in your body shape on this diet as the main criterion of success, rather than the more conventional measurement of weight loss. You will certainly lose weight (as fat) relatively quickly, but of much more significance is the way your body shape improves. This form of dieting promotes a natural body shape, which is particularly enhanced by the isometric exercise programme. It will not cause the haggard look that accompanies most calorie-control diets, because you lose fat *without* loss of the underlying body protein. You will lose fat smoothly over the body, allowing time for skin elasticity to recover, and therefore without the unsightly folds of excess skin that can occur with crash dieting. So look at your body shape as the diet progresses and watch the way that your clothes fit better, as this is a more effective measure of the diet's success than just weight loss. This type of diet has much more to offer in terms of body shape and health than the 'normal' calorie-control diet.

Drink at least four large glasses of water per day

Constipation is not a significant problem on the diet, but it can become one if you do not maintain hydration. Drink *at least* four glasses of water per day – in addition to any other drinks acceptable on the diet – and you should have no problem.

Take a multivitamin supplement

It is *very* unlikely that you will experience vitamin or mineral deficiencies on this nutritious diet (unlike many other diets). However, as a matter of safety, I always advise individuals on any diet to take a multivitamin tablet every day to ensure good health. Providing the tablet includes the daily vitamin C requirement (and most do), you no longer need to have an orange or lemon per day, saving 15 grams of daily carbohydrate intake in the process.

So now you have the knowledge to change your shape (and life) for ever, and actually have more knowledge and understanding of nutrition and health than many so-called experts, it's time for you to begin your new dietary way of life and lose weight permanently. If you have any further doubts, proceed to the delicious selection of recipes in Part II and these will be dispelled immediately.

To demonstrate how easy it is to follow the New High Protein Diet, here is a possible 2-week starter plan, but these are just suggestions. As you have seen, the beauty of this diet lies in the immense variety of foods that are included *without restriction*. On this diet, you really will eat yourself thin, and enjoy the experience.

Monday

Breakfast: 2 scrambled eggs with Parma ham
Single slice of buttered toast
Lunch: Smoked salmon and soured cream salsa
Dinner: Beef casserole with chives
Total daily carbohydrate per person: 41 grams (24 grams without toast)

Tuesday
Breakfast: Baked haddock with grilled Swiss cheese
Lunch: Omelette with filling (tomatoes/mushrooms/herbs)
Dinner: Lamb skewers with cucumber raita
Total daily carbohydrate per person:15 grams

Wednesday
Breakfast: Fried bacon, mushrooms and tomato
Lunch: Tuna mayonnaise sandwich with herbs and red pepper
             Single slice of buttered bread
Dinner: Ginger scallops with mangetout
Total daily carbohydrate per person: 30 grams (13 grams without bread)

Thursday
Breakfast: Egg mayonnaise with tomato and basil
             Single slice of buttered toast
Lunch: Chicken drumsticks
             Tomato and avocado salad
Dinner: Sliced beef in oyster sauce
             Stir-fried vegetables
Total daily carbohydrate per person: 44 grams (27 grams without toast)

Friday
Breakfast: Continental breakfast
             (sliced cheeses, ham, chicken)
             Slice of buttered bread
Lunch: Tandoori chicken
             Crispy green salad
Dinner: Trout with lemon (or lime) and pine nuts
Total daily carbohydrate per person: 43 grams (26 grams without bread)

Saturday

Breakfast: 2 eggs (poached/fried/scrambled)
Bacon and mushrooms

Lunch: Lemon sole with pak choi

Dinner: Roast duck with juniper berries and orange liqueur sauce
Carrots, mangetout and yellow squash

Total daily carbohydrate per person: 23 grams

Sunday

Breakfast: Kipper(s): one or two
Plum tomato and dill

Lunch: Roast beef
Carrots, peas

Dinner: Piperade

Total daily carbohydrate per person: 20 grams

Monday

Breakfast: Gammon steak
Tomatoes and mushrooms

Lunch: Avocado, tomato and Mozzarella sandwich (single slice of buttered bread)

Dinner: Cod with parsley sauce

Total daily carbohydrate per person: 36 grams (19 grams without bread)

Tuesday

Breakfast: 2 poached eggs with tomato
Single slice of buttered toast

Lunch: Barbecued chicken wings (from supermarket or home)
Feta salad

Dinner: Moussaka

Total carbohydrate content per person: 48 grams (31 grams without toast)

Wednesday
Breakfast: Pan-fried lemon sole
Lunch: Turkey breast with gravy
              Asparagus
Dinner: Ratatouille
Total daily carbohydrate per person: 22 grams

Thursday
Breakfast: 2 boiled eggs
              Parma ham and plum tomato
Lunch: Prawn mayonnaise sandwich
              (single slice of bread)
Dinner: Pork chops with herbs
              French beans and carrots
Total carbohydrate per person: 28 grams (11 grams without bread)

Friday
Breakfast: Toasted cheese with chives and basil
              Single slice of buttered toast
Lunch: Cod with parsley sauce
              Baby leeks
Dinner: Grilled pepper steak with French beans
Total daily carbohydrate per person: 30 grams

Saturday
Breakfast: Eggs Benedict
              ½ toasted muffin
Lunch: Mussels in garlic sauce
Dinner: Lamb's liver with mushrooms
Total daily carbohydrate per person: 35 grams (20 grams without muffin)

Sunday

Breakfast: Sliced ham and turkey
Selection of cheeses: Edam, Gruyère, Cheddar, Emmental
½ toasted muffin

Lunch: Roast lamb
Carrots and French beans

Dinner: Scallops and asparagus with sweet chilli sauce

Total daily carbohydrate per person: 30 grams (15 grams without muffin)

Before we introduce the recipes, which are both nutritious and slimming, there are a few simple principles to be outlined in the preparation and cooking of vegetables. You are probably already aware of these facts, but it's important to emphasise them as it's obviously essential to maintain as much of the nutrition and goodness in the vegetables and not lose the benefits by poor preparation and cooking techniques.

- Prepare vegetables as near the time of cooking as possible. Vegetables start to lose nutrients as soon as they are chopped, so try not to prepare vegetables in advance if possible. Obviously, however, we have to be practical. If you simply don't have time to prepare the vegetables yourself, use packs of chopped vegetables, which are readily available from supermarkets. These have lost some of the nutrients, but still provide a useful alternative in our hectic lifestyle, and are definitely better than reaching for the crisps or tin-opener.

- Lightly steam, stir-fry, or boil vegetables in as little water as possible, as this maintains the maximum nutrition.

- Never keep prepared vegetables covered with water. Nutrients leach out of vegetables quickly, and you can destroy their nutritional value by soaking them in water. Prepare vegetables at the last minute, and cook them as soon as possible.

- Add herbs and spices at every possible opportunity. Apart from the natural flavour enhancement, the nutritional benefit is immense. For example, paprika has over 10 times the vitamin A content of cabbage or green peppers, both of which are in themselves good sources of vitamin A.

- Eat the garnish! The purpose of garnish is to enhance the meal itself, not only its appearance. The garnishes utilised in these recipes are selected for both visual and nutritional content; don't leave them at the side of the plate.

- Vary the quantities in the recipes and still lose weight. The beauty of this diet is that the recipes are not cast in tablets of stone, unlike most other diets. If it is your preference to add more meat, or fish, or chicken, or vegetables, you can – without impairing the success of the diet in any way. Providing the additional ingredients are low in carbohydrate content, and you keep within your 40-gram carbohydrate limit, you can vary your menu according to taste without limits on quantities. What could be easier? All you have to do is to plan your shopping in advance, and your weight loss is assured.

- Fresh mayonnaise tastes better, but, once again,

commercial products are effective and satisfactory substitutes for the real thing. Some commercial mayonnaise even includes a significant omega-3 fatty acid component. But remember always to check the label for any undesirable ingredients.

- Many of the recipes in this book include Lebanese cucumber, which has the advantage of a lower carbohydrate content than the English variety, but obviously any cucumber will suffice.

- The recipes are usually for two people; however, the quantities of ingredients can be varied proportionately if either more or fewer people are involved: double the quantities for four, or halve for one. Bear in mind that these recipes are not just *diet* recipes, they are *normal* high-quality meals (both nutritionally and gastronomically) which may be served on any social occasion. Your can entertain guests and provide them with a healthy weight-loss diet without their knowledge! How much more considerate could you be as a host/hostess? You are caring for your guests' health and longevity, as well as their social entertainment.

PART II

Weight-Loss Phase Recipes

To kick-start your metabolism into 'weight loss mode', all of the meals you eat need to be low GI. In simple terms, this means you have to cut out all refined carbohydrates: reduce bread to a maximum of one small slice per day and no pasta, rice, cakes, chocolate, sweets or crisps, and absolutely no potatoes or parsnips. Of course, we will be reintroducing these gradually back into your diet (in moderation) after you have lost weight. This is during the subsequent 'weight-maintenance' phase (see page 227) because the aim of this system is to be a lifestyle for weight loss and health, not just another restrictive diet.

Chapter 6 Breakfast

Not many people consider having a cooked breakfast nowadays, mainly because it is considered too time-consuming. In actual fact, there is little additional time involved, and the nutritional benefits are immense. But there are still many alternatives.

Incidentally, you will notice in many of the breakfast dishes that fresh herbs are included, both for flavour and nutrition. But how are you to obtain fresh herbs every morning? Simply grow them yourself, either in the garden or in pots on the window-ledge. They are easy to grow, require little effort, cost very little to buy initially and are instantly available. The difference fresh herbs make to even the simplest of dishes is immeasurable and the cost factor insignificant.

In the following recipes you will see that I have very slightly broken some of my golden rules: occasionally you will see a little milk included in a recipe, or a teaspoon of sugar, or even a tablespoon of flour. These small quantities in a recipe for several people will make no difference to the overall carbohydrate content of the diet, and will improve the taste immensely.

Eggs

Eggs, in any form, are included to great effect, in terms of both healthy diet and gastronomic pleasure, in our breakfast menu. They are very high in protein, vitamins, minerals and anti-oxidants, with virtually no carbohydrate content, and the fat ensures a slow, even absorption of food. The potential variations on delicious recipes in which this versatile food can be used are almost limitless. Eggs will reappear in the supper section; however, in the breakfast menu I have concentrated on those dishes that can be prepared quickly.

Scrambled eggs

Scrambled eggs are probably better when cooked by the traditional method in a pan; however, this is definitely time-consuming, and may not be practical for everyone first thing in the morning. Fortunately, this dish can be quickly cooked by microwave for those who prefer. I will describe both methods and you can choose which is best for your own situation.

For 2   4 large eggs (preferably free-range)
           2 tbsp full-cream milk
           freshly ground black pepper
           25 grams butter

Traditional method

- *Break the eggs into a mixing bowl, add the milk and a little freshly ground black pepper, and beat gently with a fork to an even consistency. Melt the butter in a small pan over a low heat and add the eggs. Stir constantly, moving the edges to the middle with a circular motion, for about 2–3 minutes. Remove from heat when the eggs are no longer runny (before the eggs have set) to allow the heat of the pan to gently finish the cooking, and serve.*

By microwave

- *Add the beaten eggs to a microwave-safe bowl and place in the centre of the microwave oven. Set oven to high and cook for one minute. Remove the bowl from microwave, and stir the mixture, bringing the edges to the centre. Return to the microwave, cook on high for another minute and then stir again. Repeat the process for another minute, or until the mixture is no longer runny.*

Here are a few of the high-protein 'diet' foods that you can add to this basic recipe and continue to lose weight:

- Parma ham, finely chopped
- Smoked salmon, finely chopped
- 50 grams of grated cheese: Emmental, Jarlsberg and Gruyère are marvellous in this recipe
- 1 tbsp of fresh herbs, chopped finely and added to the mixture. Parsley, chives, basil, dill and tarragon can be added very effectively, either as individual herbs, or combined with the ingredients above
- Button mushrooms, sliced, then lightly fried in a little butter
- Plum tomatoes (two), seeded and diced
- Bacon rasher, diced finely and lightly fried in butter

*Carbohydrate content per serving: **2–3** grams, depending on added ingredients*

Eggs are one of the very few foods which I consider it is almost impossible to enjoy without bread (our forbidden carbohydrate); however, restrict yourself to one slice of buttered wholemeal toast (which equates to 17 grams of carbohydrate in itself).

Omelette

For 2   4 large eggs (preferably free-range)
freshly ground black pepper
pinch of rock salt
2 tbsp full-cream milk
25 grams butter

• *Whisk the eggs, seasoning and milk with a fork to an even consistency. Melt the butter in an omelette pan (or small frying pan), tilting the pan to ensure an even coating of butter. When the butter is hot but not burning, add the egg mixture. Stir the mixture with the fork until the omelette sets, then stop stirring. Cook the omelette for about another minute, then, using a palette knife, gently lift one edge of the omelette, fold one half over the other and slide the omelette onto a plate.*

Omelettes can be an ideal meal for breakfast, brunch, lunch, dinner, or supper, depending on the occasion and the time available for preparation. They can be as simple or as complicated as you wish. The fillings described for scrambled eggs (such as Parma ham, smoked salmon, cheeses, herbs, tomatoes, mushrooms and bacon) are equally suitable for omelettes.

Frittata, an Italian modification of the French omelette, takes a little longer to prepare as it involves cooking the eggs more thoroughly to produce a more solid end-product. As the typical frittata takes 15 minutes of slow cooking, it may not be suitable for weekday breakfast. However, it can, of course, be prepared the previous evening and provide the perfect 'instant' nutritious breakfast. As frittata takes longer to cook, I have included it in the lunch/dinner section (see pages 186–7, 188).

Carbohydrate content per serving: 2–3 grams (depending on added ingredients)

Boiled eggs

For 2   2 large free-range eggs

- *Probably the only meal that is even faster than opening the cereal packet! Place 2 large eggs in warm water, bring to the boil, then reduce the heat to a gentle simmer. Excessive boiling will spoil the flavour and often causes the eggs to crack. The length of simmering depends on how you prefer your boiled eggs: with large eggs, between 3 minutes for soft-boiled to 8 minutes for hard-boiled.*

In my opinion, boiled eggs are impossible to enjoy without toast, but again restrict yourself to one slice of buttered wholemeal toast per person. Or you can hard boil the eggs and enjoy them with some finely sliced Emmental or Jarlsberg cheese, perhaps with some slices of Parma ham or finely sliced turkey breast. These latter ingredients sound expensive, but they are not. If you buy some cheese and a packet of sliced ham or chicken breast from the delicatessen, a little each day is actually very inexpensive. The restriction of carbohydrate in this diet decreases appetite to a normal level and reduces cravings for large quantities of food. In that respect, the diet is self-sustaining.

Carbohydrate content per serving: negligible (without toast); 17 grams (with toast)

Poached eggs
For 2   2 large free-range eggs

Once again, the wonders of modern science allow us to poach eggs either by the traditional method or more rapidly by microwave, which, while it may not seem very trendy, is immensely beneficial to those hard-pressed for time in the morning.

Traditional method
   • *Heat the water to boiling point in a shallow pan, then reduce the heat to a gentle simmer. Break each egg individually into a cup, and slide the eggs gently into the boiling water. Cook for approximately 3–4 minutes, removing the eggs from the water with a perforated spoon when the yolk is evenly coated with a white film and the white has cooked. Serve on a slice of buttered wholemeal toast.*

By microwave
   • *Break each egg individually into the plastic cups specially designed for microwave poaching of eggs. Pierce the top of the yolks four to five times with a sharp knife, add a teaspoon of cold water and close the sealed top of the cup. Cook on medium (careful, on high it will explode!) for about 1–2 minutes (depending on the power of the microwave), then allow to stand for another minute before serving.*

Carbohydrate content per serving: negligible (without toast); 17 grams (with toast)

Eggs Benedict

The classic recipe includes Canadian bacon; however, this version incorporates prosciutto for a lighter flavour. The lemon hollandaise sauce can be prepared the previous day.

For 2
2 large free-range eggs, poached
1 English muffin
50 grams prosciutto
hollandaise sauce (see page 110)
chopped fresh chives, to garnish

- *Prepare the hollandaise sauce according to the recipe on page 110 but use only 1 teaspoon of lemon juice. Halve the muffin and toast each half lightly. Lay the prosciutto on each half muffin. Poach the eggs, place the drained poached eggs on the ham and top with hollandaise sauce, garnished with chopped chives.*

Carbohydrate content per serving: **15** *grams (including muffin)*

Fish

Fish is not a common breakfast dish today, but that is merely a reflection of modern society. It was not so very long ago that fish was one of the staple dishes on the breakfast menu, and there is really no reason why it should not continue to be. It is the original fast food, with the difference that it is full of virtually every kind of goodness you can imagine: protein, essential fatty acids, vitamins, minerals, natural antioxidants and virtually no carbohydrate. And the dishes can be as simple or as complicated as time will allow. For breakfast I am going to concentrate on dishes which are relatively quick and simple to prepare. Some of the more time-consuming fish recipes are described later, but of course the choice is yours.

Pan-fried lemon sole
This is one of life's simple pleasures, and it could not be more delicious. In my opinion, it is a suitable meal at any time of day.

For 2
2 lemon sole fillets
60 grams butter
lemon wedges
1 tsp chopped fresh basil
2 tsp freshly squeezed lemon juice
freshly ground black pepper

- *Heat the butter in the pan and sauté the lemon sole fillets, for about 1–1½ minutes per side, turning carefully once with a fish slice. Serve the fillets onto warm plates. Add the basil to the butter in the pan, stir in the lemon juice, and heat gently for a few seconds. Pour the sauce over the fish, season to taste and serve with lemon wedges.*
- *The fillets can be dusted with flour if you prefer; however, with careful cooking – and in particular the use of a fish slice – they will not break up, and flour really doesn't add anything to the flavour. The avoidance of any unnecessary carbohydrate in the diet is a definite advantage.*
- *Cod or haddock can substitute for lemon sole, but the larger fillets take longer, and are not as suitable for rapid cooking at breakfast.*

*Carbohydrate content per serving: **1** gram*

Baked haddock with grilled Swiss cheese

For 2   2 haddock fillets
100 ml full-cream milk
1 tbsp chopped fresh chives
1 tbsp chopped fresh basil
50 grams grated Emmental cheese
freshly ground black pepper

- *If you have just a few extra moments to spare in the morning, this baked haddock recipe is delightful.*
- *Place the haddock fillet in an oven-safe dish and add the full-cream milk and the chopped fresh herbs. Cover with pierced aluminium foil, and cook at 190 degrees C (gas mark 4) for 20 minutes.*
- *Drain the haddock and place it on a slice of hot, buttered wholemeal toast. Grate some Emmental cheese over the haddock and place under a hot grill for 30–40 seconds.*
- *The Emmental can be replaced by Gruyère, Jarlsberg or Edam (the latter are certainly not Swiss cheeses, but are equally suitable for this delicious recipe) according to your personal preference. I consider Cheddar cheese a little too overpowering for haddock.*

*Carbohydrate content per serving: **3** grams (**20** grams including toast)*

Poached eggs and smoked haddock

For 2 2 small smoked haddock fillets
1 bay leaf
pinch of rock salt
2 large free-range eggs
freshly ground black pepper
2 slices buttered wholemeal toast (optional)

- *Place the smoked haddock fillets in a deep frying pan, add hot water to just cover the fillets, then add the bay leaf and a pinch of rock salt. Bring to the boil and reduce the heat to a gentle simmer for about 3–4 minutes. In a medium saucepan, poach the eggs to taste (see page 72). Transfer the cooked haddock fillets carefully with a fish slice to separate warm plates and place a poached egg on each haddock fillet. Add some freshly ground black pepper, and serve with a slice of buttered wholemeal toast (optional).*

Carbohydrate content per serving: negligible (17 grams with toast)

Kippers

Kippers are among the world's great dishes – on their own!
Sauces and accompaniments to dishes are the prerogative of
many great gastronomic nations, but the Europeans have
wonderful foods with natural taste, either directly from the sea,
or manufactured by some of the greatest cheese-makers in the
world.

The North Sea provides us with natural foods full of natural
flavour; however, some enterprising and brilliant innovators in
gastronomic cuisine – many hundreds (and possibly thousands)
of years before the word 'cuisine' was in current usage –
managed actually to improve on the natural taste of the fish by
smoking it in a way that has remained unchanged (because it
probably cannot be improved).

Kippers can be cooked in many ways, but the two easiest –
and quickest – are frying and poaching. Both are almost
equally rapid, equally nutritious and equally tasty. The only
difference is individual preference.

Fried kipper

For 1   1 kipper
          60 grams butter
          1 plum tomato, diced
          1 tbsp chopped fresh dill
          freshly ground black pepper
          1 slice buttered wholemeal toast (optional)

- *Heat the butter in a shallow frying pan, add the kipper
  and cook for 2 minutes on each side. Season to
  taste, garnish with chopped tomato and fresh dill, and
  serve with a slice of buttered wholemeal toast. The
  toast may be omitted if you wish to reduce your daily
  carbohydrates.*

*Carbohydrate content per serving: **3** grams (**20** grams
with toast)*

Mushrooms

Mushrooms are a magnificent source of vitamin B, they taste wonderful (either alone or with fresh herbs) and they are quick and simple to prepare and cook. So unless you actually dislike mushrooms, remember to include *fresh* mushrooms in your diet. Mushrooms are equally enjoyable for breakfast, lunch, supper or dinner – or even as a late-night snack.

Mushrooms on toast

Simple title, simple preparation, but a delicious, rapid and nutritious breakfast.

The flavour (but not the nutritional value) can vary dramatically with the type of mushroom used. I will describe a simple recipe with button mushrooms, but I would advise you experiment with various types of mushrooms to discover which flavour you prefer; mushrooms – like fish and cheese – are very much a case of individual preference, but all are equally nutritious, so you simply can't get it wrong. Button mushrooms are particularly useful in dieting as they have the same vitamin content but lower carbohydrate content than other varieties of mushroom.

For 2
150 grams button mushrooms
50 grams butter
1 tbsp chopped chives
1 tbsp chopped basil
pinch of rock salt
pinch of paprika (optional)
freshly ground black pepper
2 slices buttered wholemeal toast

- *Clean the mushrooms by wiping them carefully, and remove the lower half-centimetre from the base of each stalk. Cut the button mushrooms in half lengthways. Heat the butter in a medium saucepan, and add the mushrooms. Cook for about 2 minutes, stirring frequently, then add the herbs, salt and paprika. Season to taste and cook for a further 2 minutes. Remove the mushroom and herb mixture with a perforated spoon and serve on warm plates with buttered wholemeal toast.*

Carbohydrate content per serving: *1 gram (18 grams with toast)*

For the cook in a hurry in the morning, an even easier – and just as tasty and nutritious – mushroom breakfast can be prepared as follows.

For 2
2 large flat mushrooms
50 grams butter
2 plum tomatoes, diced
1 tbsp chopped fresh coriander
pinch of rock salt
freshly ground black pepper
2 slices buttered wholemeal toast

- *Dice a plum tomato, mix with a little chopped fresh coriander, cover and set aside.*
- *Wipe the mushrooms and trim the base of the stalks. Heat the butter in a shallow frying pan, sauté the mushrooms for approximately 2–3 minutes per side (depending on thickness), turning once, and serve on a slice of buttered wholemeal toast. Top with the tomato and coriander mixture, and season with freshly ground black pepper. Simple, nutritious, delicious and slimming!*

Carbohydrate content per serving: *2 grams (19 grams with toast)*

Cheese

One of the nice things about using high-protein, low-carbohydrate foods is that they are so adaptable and yet they all taste delicious on their own: meat, poultry, fish, eggs and cheese – the original fast food.

Don't pigeon-hole cheese into a snack or dessert food. Apart from last thing at night (when there are definite medical reasons for not eating it), cheese is adaptable to every meal-time. Breakfast is no exception.

Toasted cheese

Toasted cheese for breakfast can be served alone or with delicious accompaniments which are relatively inexpensive (in the small quantities involved) and yet quick to prepare and serve. This meal is limited only by your preference in cheese, because the almost unlimited variety of cheeses can provide a different breakfast every day of the year. Cheddar cheese is excellent for this purpose; however, for variety try Edam, Gouda, Emmental, Gruyère or Jarlsberg – or whichever cheese you prefer.

For 2
2 slices buttered wholemeal bread
grated cheese (Cheddar, Edam, Gouda, Emmental, Gruyère or Jarlsberg)
freshly ground black pepper

- *Lightly toast one side of a slice of wholemeal bread, then remove from the grill. Add grated cheese to the non-toasted side and return to the grill until the cheese has melted.*
- *Add some freshly ground black pepper, then serve alone or with a little pickle.*

For variety, freshly grated cheese can be mixed with the following additional ingredients before toasting, to provide a truly delicious breakfast:

- Parma ham, finely diced
- plum tomato, diced
- ¼ red pepper, deseeded and diced
- spring onion, finely chopped
- 1 tbsp chopped fresh chives and basil
- ¼ green chilli, deseeded and finely chopped
- 1 tsp of Worcester sauce and 2 drops of Tabasco sauce
- finely diced smoked salmon and 1 tsp chopped dill

Heaven on toast!

Carbohydrate content per serving: **17–18** grams (including the toast)

Continental breakfast

This is a term which covers a multitude of sins, but in this context it is taken to mean a cold platter, easily and quickly prepared to provide a nutritious meal with virtually no carbohydrate content, and therefore ideal for the serious slimmer. Cheeses; slices of cold ham, chicken or turkey; boiled eggs; an orange (but no other fruit at the early stage in the diet); and a slice of buttered wholemeal bread or toast (optional) are all included, but definitely no croissants, pastries, jams or marmalade.

Chapter 7 Lunch on the run

Lunches may be simply divided into those that are made for us (take-aways and restaurant meals) and those we prepare ourselves (packed lunches and meals at home). The difference is important when we are dieting to lose fat. Let's look at the various categories separately and see how easy it is to apply the principles of a low-carbohydrate diet to each situation.

Take-away

In most cases the term 'fast food' is merely a synonym for 'high-carbohydrate food', which is disastrous for an effective diet. Avoid chips, burgers, pies, quiche, pasta, pitta, rice and any of the other obvious sources of unwanted carbohydrates. Shish kebabs can be included – providing you have very little bread or pitta. Pre-packed sandwiches are acceptable, but be careful: keep to the restriction of only one slice of bread per day and make sure the fillings comply with our carbohydrate restriction guidelines. You can have an unlimited amount of tuna mayonnaise or prawn mayonnaise on the sandwich, but only one slice of bread. Certainly no cakes or pastries – but then, you knew that already!

Remember the other forms of take-away which are less obvious: the supermarkets for example. These outlets provide many forms of take-away foods which are eminently suitable to be included in a low-carbohydrate diet:

- chicken drumsticks and chicken wings (plain and with sauces, such as barbecue, tikka and Chinese)
- gourmet ham
- Chinese chicken and breast fillets
- calamari
- smoked salmon

The list is almost endless. Check the carbohydrate content of the various foods and you will see that many pre-prepared fast foods in supermarkets are actually low in carbohydrates and therefore 'diet-friendly'.

Restaurant meals

If you intend to eat at a restaurant, choose meat, fish, poultry or pork *without* sauces. At home you can prepare sauces very effectively without sugar (and with a lesser amount of flour), but restaurants may not do so, therefore sauces are best avoided, as hidden sugars can completely ruin your carbohydrate restriction and thereby ruin your diet. Providing you didn't have eggs for breakfast, eggs (cooked any way you like) are fine, as is mayonnaise. Add salad, vegetables without sauces (obviously no potatoes) or herbs to the main course without restriction. On these minimal restrictions, the choice in restaurant menus is immense.

Packed lunches

Packed lunches can be exciting or simple, depending upon the time you have available for preparation, but need never be boring, even if you have limited preparation time. Good food needs little preparation because it has its own natural flavours: what could taste better than the plethora of cheeses available, meat, poultry, fish, seafood and vegetables?

Sandwiches

You can, of course, prepare your own sanwiches as part of a daily carbohydrate restriction diet. In other words, no more than *one* slice of wholemeal bread per day (in the early stages of the diet). This restriction can be increased to two slices per day later in the diet, but obviously if you decide on a sandwich for lunch, you can't have any toast for breakfast. The important principle of this diet is to restrict carbohydrates; break the rule – even once – and you're back to square one for that particular day. You can eat as much as you want of the unrestricted foods and still lose weight *only providing you keep your carbohydrate intake below 40–60 grams per day.* If you eat more carbohydrate, the insulin mechanism is stimulated and the other foods in your diet (fats and protein) are working *against* you – instead of *for* you – by being converted into body fat.

Fillings for a sandwich need not be restricted to the standard diet fare, which is usually some form of salad – without mayonnaise, or with French dressing (*sans* sugar). The only restriction in this diet is carbohydrate content, not calories. So ensure that you butter the bread (or use margarine if you prefer), both for the vitamins in butter and the slowing of the digestion provided by the lipid content of the butter. All of these sandwiches can be prepared either as closed sandwiches or – even better – as open sandwiches. Providing the fillings are low in carbohydrate, the possibilities are almost endless, but you have to restrict yourself to only one slice of wholemeal bread per day. Previously, you were told to restrict calories, but now you have to learn to think in the opposite way: you have to restrict carbohydrate content – so sandwich fillings are largely unrestricted, but the bread becomes the problem. On the next two pages is a selection of wonderful fillings which are entirely commensurate with a successful slimming diet.

Sandwich fillings

Avocado

For 2
1 small ripe Hass avocado, halved, peeled, stoned and finely sliced *with*
either diced plum tomato or sliced Mozzarella cheese or both
2 slices buttered wholemeal bread
1 tbsp extra-virgin olive oil
2 tsp balsamic vinegar
freshly ground black pepper

- *Arrange the sliced avocado on a slice of buttered wholemeal bread. Top with either diced plum tomato or sliced Mozzarella cheese (or both). Drizzle the extra-virgin olive oil and balsamic vinegar over the filling and season with freshly ground black pepper.*

Carbohydrate content per serving: 3 grams (20 grams with bread)

Salad

If you prefer gourmet salad sandwiches for lunch, rather than the usual wet lettuce and tomato, try the following, and still lose weight:

- Feta salad (page 205)
- Bocconcini and avocado salad (page 206)
- tomato and Mozzarella salad (page 210)
- cucumber and bean sprout salad (page 211)
- tomato salsa (page 225)

But remember, only one slice of bread per day. So if you intend to have a sandwich for lunch, don't have toast with breakfast.

Chicken

There are so many different ways to use chicken in sandwiches that I can only briefly scrape the surface of possibilities here, but a few delicious ideas follow. On a practical level, unless you have more available time than most of us in the morning, it is easier to cook the chicken the previous evening, although obviously chicken does taste better freshly cooked. If there is no time to cook the chicken the previous evening, you can substitute sliced turkey or chicken breast from either a delicatessen or supermarket. Remember, while we are trying to make these meals as tasty as possible, they have to be practical for the modern world, because if you can't adhere to the diet, it won't work – which is the basic fault of most diets!

Chicken with mayonnaise and avocado

For 2   1 small chicken breast fillet
2 tbsp extra-virgin olive oil
1 tbsp mayonnaise
half a small ripe Hass avocado, finely sliced
2 slices buttered wholemeal bread
freshly ground black pepper

- *Sauté the chicken fillet in the olive oil for approximately 5 minutes on each side, turning once, until cooked. Set aside to cool, then slice finely. Mix with the mayonnaise and spoon on to a slice of buttered wholemeal bread. Arrange the avocado slices on the chicken and season with freshly ground black pepper.*

*Carbohydrate content per serving: **1** gram (**18** grams with bread)*

Chicken with Swiss cheese

For 2   1 small chicken breast fillet
2 tbsp extra-virgin olive oil
2 slices buttered wholemeal bread
1 tbsp tomato salsa (see page 225)
50 grams grated Emmental cheese
freshly ground black pepper

- *Prepare the tomato salsa according to the recipe on page 225. This can obviously be done the day before.*
- *Sauté the chicken, as described overleaf, chop into cubes and arrange on a slice of buttered wholemeal bread. Spoon the tomato salsa on the chicken and add some freshly ground black pepper. Top with grated cheese of your choice. (I prefer Emmental or Jarlsberg for this sandwich, but cheese is such an individual taste that virtually any will suffice – with the possible exception of Cheddar, which I personally find too overpowering a flavour for chicken.)*
- *This can be served cold, as either an open or closed sandwich, or the open sandwich can be modified by placing it under a hot grill until the cheese has melted, to provide a delicious hot open sandwich.*

*Carbohydrate content per serving: **4** grams (**21** grams with bread)*

Tuna

Tuna has the marvellous advantage over most of its fast-but-nutritious food rivals that it is instantly available from a tin, and the tinned variety retains its nutritional value entirely – the quintessential pre-packed food (almost unique in this respect). The only disadvantage with tuna is . . . there isn't any! It's a perfect ingredient in any healthy diet – whether you need to lose weight or not.

For 2
200-gram tin of tuna (in brine or springwater), drained
1 tbsp mayonnaise
1 tbsp chopped fresh basil
1 tsp chopped fresh coriander
freshly ground black pepper
2 slices buttered wholemeal bread
1 vine-ripened tomato, diced (optional)
½ small red pepper, deseeded and sliced thinly
    (optional)
1 tsp chopped fresh chives

- Flake the tuna and mix with the mayonnaise, chopped basil and coriander, and freshly ground black pepper. Spoon the mixture liberally on two slices of buttered wholemeal bread. This is delicious alone, or add diced vine-ripened tomato (and/or sliced red pepper with chopped fresh chives) for extra flavour and nutrition.

*Carbohydrate content per serving: **2** grams (**19** grams with bread)*

Lunches prepared at home

Lunches can be prepared at home either as a packed lunch to go or as a meal to be eaten at home. The only real difference between lunch, supper, dinner and late snacks is the size of the meal relative to the time of day; therefore you should look at the following chapters for at-home lunch recipes. The possible variations are infinite – from salmon with lemon butter (see pages 102–3) to prosciutto and courgette frittata (see page 186).

In this book you will notice a significant preponderance of stir-frying. This is a very healthy method of cooking and I cannot recommend it strongly enough. The ingredients are finely sliced, ensuring rapid cooking in a very short period, thereby retaining both the flavour and the nutritional value of the food. And there is the added advantage of a single pan to clean at the end of the meal. Simply perfect!

Chapter 8 Soups

Avocado soup

For 2

50 grams butter
1 medium onion, peeled and diced
1 garlic clove, peeled and finely chopped
1 tbsp plain flour
250 ml chicken stock
1 large, ripe Hass avocado, halved, stoned, peeled
   and chopped
1 tbsp freshly squeezed lemon juice
pinch of rock salt
freshly ground black pepper
60 ml single cream

- *Heat the butter in a medium frying pan and sauté the onion and garlic for 1–2 minutes. Remove from the heat and add the flour, mixing well. Gradually stir in the chicken stock, to ensure an even consistency. Cook over a low heat for 3–4 minutes.*

- *Add the avocado, lemon juice and chicken stock mixture to a blender and purée. Season to taste, add almost all of the cream and blend until smooth. Either chill for 1–2 hours and serve cool, or return to a clean saucepan and heat gently through – without boiling. This soup is definitely ruined by overcooking. Pour into bowls and add a swirl of cream before serving.*

*Carbohydrate content per serving: **4** grams*

Tomato and basil soup

For 2   2 tbsp extra-virgin olive oil
350 grams plum tomatoes, peeled and chopped
1 garlic clove, peeled and finely chopped
3 spring onions, finely chopped
2 tbsp chopped fresh basil
1 bay leaf
350 ml chicken (or vegetable) stock
1 tbsp tomato purée
freshly ground black pepper
2 tsp cornflour
100 ml single cream
pinch of rock salt
2 tsp chopped fresh basil to garnish

- *Cut a shallow cross through the skin of each tomato at its base and place in a bowl of boiling water for 30 seconds, then drain. Immerse the tomatoes in cold water for a few seconds, then the skin should peel easily.*
- *Heat the olive oil in a large saucepan, then add the tomatoes, garlic and spring onions, and cook for 2–3 minutes, stirring frequently. Add the basil, bay leaf, stock and tomato purée. Season with freshly ground black pepper, but do not add further salt at this stage as the stock may be quite salty. Bring to the boil and simmer for 20–30 minutes, then sieve the mixture into a clean saucepan. Make the cornflour into an even paste with a little cold water and add to the soup, mixing evenly. Stir over a low heat until the soup thickens. Add salt to taste. Stir in the cream and serve garnished with chopped basil.*

*Carbohydrate content per serving: **20** grams*

Hot pepper and coriander soup

Perfect served hot for a cold winter's evening, or chilled as a starter.

For 2
2 tbsp extra-virgin olive oil
1 large red pepper, deseeded and diced
1 large red chilli, deseeded and finely chopped
1 garlic clove, peeled and finely chopped
½ tsp ground turmeric
½ tsp ground cumin
3 curry leaves
400 ml tomato juice
2 tsp tomato purée
1 tbsp chopped fresh coriander
1 tbsp freshly squeezed lemon juice
pinch of rock salt
freshly ground black pepper
chopped fresh chives, to garnish

- *Heat the olive oil and sauté the pepper, chilli and garlic for about a minute. Add the ground turmeric, cumin and curry leaves, and cook for a further minute. Stir in the tomato juice, tomato purée, chopped coriander and lemon juice. Season to taste and simmer for 15–20 minutes. Remove the curry leaves, and serve immediately, garnished with chopped fresh chives.*

*Carbohydrate content per serving: **12** grams*

Carrot and coriander soup

For 2   2 tbsp extra-virgin olive oil
         1 medium onion, peeled and finely diced
         1 garlic clove, peeled and finely chopped
         200 grams carrots, finely grated
         400 ml chicken stock
         1 tbsp chopped fresh coriander
         2 tsp freshly squeezed lemon juice
         pinch of rock salt (optional)
         freshly ground black pepper
         100 ml single cream
         2 tsp chopped fresh chives, to garnish

- *Heat the olive oil in a medium saucepan and sauté the onion and garlic for about a minute. Add the carrots, mixing well, and sauté on a very low heat for 6–8 minutes. Stir in the chicken stock and coriander. Add the lemon juice, season to taste and simmer for 25–30 minutes. This soup can be puréed; however, I prefer the chunky variety. Stir in the cream and serve immediately, garnished with chopped chives.*

Carbohydrate content per serving: **9** *grams*

Cream of chicken soup

For 2   50 grams unsalted butter
1 medium onion, peeled and finely diced
1 garlic clove, peeled and finely chopped
1 medium carrot, finely grated
350 ml chicken stock
150 grams cooked skinless chicken breast, finely
   chopped
pinch of rock salt
freshly ground black pepper
1 tbsp chopped fresh chives
1 tbsp chopped fresh basil
150 ml single cream
2 tsp chopped fresh basil leaves, to garnish

- *Heat the butter in a medium saucepan and sauté the
  onion and garlic for about a minute. Stir in the grated
  carrot and sauté for a further 2–3 minutes. Add the
  chicken stock and chopped chicken, season to taste
  and simmer for about 15 minutes. Add the chives
  and basil, and blend in a processor until smooth. This
  can be set aside until required. Immediately before
  serving, stir in the cream and gently heat through,
  stirring constantly, but do not allow to boil. Serve
  immediately, garnished with chopped fresh basil.*

Carbohydrate content per serving: **5** *grams*

Carrot and orange soup

For 2   50 grams unsalted butter
1 medium onion, peeled and finely diced
200 grams carrots, finely grated
500 ml chicken stock
1 tbsp fresh chopped basil
½ tsp ground nutmeg
juice of a freshly squeezed orange
pinch of rock salt
freshly ground black pepper
2 tbsp single cream

* *Heat the butter in a medium saucepan and sauté the onion for 2–3 minutes. Stir in the carrots and cook for 4–5 minutes on very low heat. Add the chicken stock, chopped basil, nutmeg and orange juice, and season to taste. Simmer gently for 20–30 minutes and serve, adding a swirl of fresh cream.*

*Carbohydrate content per serving: **15** grams*

Gazpacho

For 2   1 medium red pepper, deseeded and chopped
1 medium green pepper, deseeded and chopped
1 large green chilli, deseeded and finely chopped
1 garlic clove, peeled and finely chopped
1 Lebanese cucumber, chopped
1 medium red onion, peeled and chopped
400 grams ripe plum tomatoes, peeled and chopped
2 tbsp red wine vinegar
3 tbsp extra-virgin olive oil
300 ml unsweetened tomato juice
2 tsp chopped fresh basil
pinch of rock salt
freshly ground black pepper

- *Before commencing, set aside a little of the chopped red and green peppers, cucumber, onion and chilli – sufficient for garnish later.*
- *Blend the peppers, cucumber, onion, chilli, garlic, tomatoes, red wine vinegar, olive oil and tomato juice in a food processor. Season to taste and chill for at least 2 hours in the fridge. Serve chilled, garnished with the chopped peppers, cucumber, onion and red chilli.*

*Carbohydrate content per serving: **27** grams*

Chilled cucumber soup

For 2   1 large cucumber, peeled and diced
300 ml vegetable stock
2 tbsp chopped fresh chives
1 tbsp chopped fresh basil leaves
freshly ground black pepper
150 ml single cream

- *Place the cucumber and stock in a large saucepan, bring to the boil and simmer gently for about 30 minutes.*
- *Stir in 1 tablespoon of chopped fresh chives and the basil leaves and season to taste. Transfer to a blender and mix until smooth.*
- *Return the soup to the pan, stir in the cream and heat through gently for about 2–3 minutes.*
- *Transfer the mixture to a medium bowl and chill in the fridge for at least 2 hours.*
- *Serve garnished with chopped chives.*

*Carbohydrate content per serving: **8** grams*

Smoked haddock soup

For 2

50 grams butter
1 large brown onion, peeled and diced
2 large leeks, topped and tailed and sliced
    lengthways into 5-cm segments
1 garlic clove, peeled and grated
2 slices root ginger, peeled and diced
500 ml fish stock
300 grams undyed smoked haddock fillet, chopped
    into large chunks
100 ml double cream
freshly ground black pepper
1 tbsp chopped fresh coriander leaves

- *Melt the butter in a large saucepan and sauté the onion, leeks, garlic and ginger for 2–3 minutes.*
- *Stir in the fish stock and the haddock.*
- *Bring to the boil and then simmer for approximately 7–10 minutes.*
- *Stir in the cream and season to taste.*
- *Garnish with chopped fresh coriander leaves and serve immediately.*

*Carbohydrate content per serving: **10** grams*

Chapter **9** Fish

Fish can be successfully served at virtually any time of day – from breakfast to supper – and is an essential part of any healthy diet, irrespective of whether you need to lose weight or not. We have already dealt (very briefly) with some possible fish recipes for breakfast. At lunch, we can be a little more adventurous, though obviously time is a constraint on all meals before dinner. Perhaps the easiest – and lightest – dishes are salmon and trout; they are certainly among the richest and most delicious fish on their own merits, and are quite inexpensive in real terms, especially when you consider that you require relatively small portions per person of these rich dishes, and the nutritional value is excellent.

Salmon

Salmon is the perfect meal, with just a simple sauce or salad to enhance its rich flavour. Because it is a fish full of natural oils, it loses none of its flavour by grilling.

Grilled salmon

For 1   1 salmon steak (approximately 2–2.5 cm thick)
       1 tbsp extra-virgin olive oil

- *Brush both sides of the steak with a little olive oil and grill under a hot grill for 3–4 minutes per side, turning once. Serve immediately with either lightly steamed mangetout or a simple fresh salad, for example rocket and avocado salad (page 213).*

*Carbohydrate content per serving: **2** grams*

Poached salmon

Whilst it is quite acceptable to grill rich oily fish, such as salmon, I prefer to retain its delicate flavour and texture by poaching or baking, which I cannot help but believe also retains the nutritional value better than the rather harsher environment of the grill tray. In any event, salmon is equally simple to cook by either method. Allow one salmon steak of about 150 grams per person.

In a saucepan boil sufficient water to just cover the salmon steaks, then reduce the heat to a gentle simmer. Add a pinch of salt to the water, then lay the fillets in the base of the pan *gently*, and cook for 4–5 minutes. Remove with a fish slice to prevent flaking of the fish, drain and serve on a warm plate with a simple sauce, such as lemon butter sauce (see below).

In the Southern hemisphere, the salmon tends to have a light texture, but a rather bland flavour, and therefore requires sauces for flavour enhancement. However, in the Northern hemisphere, seafood of all varieties has strong and distinctive flavours, and sauces must be light to complement the intrinsic piquancy of the seafood. Salmon has such a rich natural flavour that it requires only the addition of freshly squeezed lemon or lime juice, or a simple lemon and herb butter sauce to complement and accentuate its unique taste to perfection. Several herbs seem to have been developed in nature essentially to accompany fresh salmon!

Lightly steamed (to retain the nutritional value) mangetout or sugar snap peas with yellow squash will complement the flavour and colour of the salmon admirably – with virtually no additional carbohydrate.

Lemon butter sauce

For 2   60 grams unsalted butter
juice from ½ a freshly squeezed lemon

- *Heat the butter in a small saucepan and stir in the freshly squeezed lemon juice. Simmer for 20–30 seconds and serve over the salmon steaks.*

Carbohydrate content per serving: **2** grams

Lemon and dill butter sauce

For 2   60 grams unsalted butter
juice from ½ a freshly squeezed lemon
2 tbsp chopped fresh dill

- *Prepare as above, but add 2 tbsp of chopped fresh dill with the juice of the lemon to the butter, simmer for 30 seconds and serve over the salmon steaks.*

Carbohydrate content per serving: **2** grams

Lemon and basil butter sauce

For 2   60 grams unsalted butter
juice from ½ a freshly squeezed lemon
2 tbsp chopped fresh basil

- *Prepare as above, substituting 2 tbsp of chopped fresh basil leaves for the dill.*

Carbohydrate content per serving: **2** grams

Smoked salmon and soured cream salsa

For 2   4 leaves of radicchio lettuce, washed
1 small smoked salmon fillet, sliced finely on the
   diagonal
pinch of paprika and some fresh basil leaves, to
   garnish

Sour cream salsa

100 ml soured cream
½ Lebanese cucumber, peeled. Cut 2 slices from the
   cucumber, then chop the remainder into small cubes
1 tbsp chopped fresh basil
freshly ground black pepper

- *Mix together the soured cream, chopped cucumber and chopped basil, season with freshly ground black pepper, and set aside to chill in the fridge for 1–2 hours.*
- *Arrange 2 leaves of radicchio lettuce on each plate. Place a slice of cucumber in the centre of the lettuce, and arrange several strips of smoked salmon on the cucumber slice. Spoon a tablespoon of soured cream salsa on the smoked salmon, then add a second layer of smoked salmon and top with another tablespoon of soured cream salsa. Sprinkle with a pinch of paprika and some fresh basil leaves to garnish, and serve immediately or chill in the fridge until required.*

*Carbohydrate content per serving: **3** grams*

Salmon pâté

I have suggested quantities sufficient for four people in this recipe, as it tastes equally delicious the next day for breakfast or lunch.

For 4
    25 grams butter
    1 medium onion, peeled and finely diced
    1 garlic clove, peeled and finely chopped
    200-gram tin of red salmon, bones removed, drained and flaked
    1 tbsp freshly squeezed lemon juice
    1 tbsp dry sherry
    1 tbsp chopped fresh flat-leaf parsley
    1 large free-range egg, beaten
    2 tbsp fine toasted breadcrumbs
    50 grams butter, melted
    pinch of rock salt
    freshly ground black pepper
    lemon wedges
    sprigs of fresh flat-leaf parsley, to garnish

- *Heat butter in a small saucepan and sauté the onion and garlic until softened. Transfer the onion and garlic to a large mixing bowl, add the salmon, then stir in the lemon juice, sherry, chopped parsley, egg, breadcrumbs and melted butter. Season to taste and mix thoroughly. Line a loaf tin with aluminium foil and press the salmon pâté mixture firmly in the base of the tin.*
- *Close the foil parcel loosely and cook in the centre of a pre-heated oven at 180 degrees C (gas mark 4) for 45 minutes. Remove and set aside to cool. Serve with a crispy green salad (page 209) and lemon wedges, garnished with sprigs of fresh flat-leaf parsley.*

*Carbohydrate content per serving: **16** grams*

Chilli salmon kebabs

For 2   2 tbsp chilli sauce
juice from ½ a freshly squeezed lemon
300 grams skinless salmon fillets, cut into large
   segments
extra-virgin olive oil
coriander leaves to garnish
freshly ground black pepper

- Mix together the chilli sauce and lemon juice.
- Marinate the salmon in the chilli and lemon for approximately 1 hour.
- Thread the salmon segments on to skewers, drizzle with a little extra-virgin olive oil and cook for 4 minutes on each side on a griddle.
- Serve immediately, garnished with fresh coriander leaves and seasoned with black pepper.

*Carbohydrate content per serving: **10** grams*

Spicy salmon

For 2   2 fresh salmon fillets, approximately 150 grams each
butter
1 tbsp extra-virgin olive oil
1 garlic clove, peeled and diced
2 slices of fresh ginger, peeled and finely chopped
1 small green chilli, deseeded and finely chopped
100 grams rocket leaves
100 grams baby spinach leaves
50 ml Sauvignon Blanc
1 tbsp light soy sauce
fresh flat-leaf parsley, to garnish
thin strips of fresh red chilli, to garnish

- Place the salmon fillets in a roasting tin, dot with butter and cover with perforated aluminium foil.
- Cook in the centre of a preheated oven at 180 degrees C (gas mark 4) for 18–20 minutes.
- Remove the salmon from the oven and set aside.

At the same time
- *Heat the extra-virgin olive oil in a wok, and stir-fry the garlic, ginger and chilli for about 30–40 seconds.*
- *Add the rocket and spinach and stir-fry for 30 seconds.*
- *Stir in the Sauvignon Blanc.*
- *Add the soy sauce and stir-fry until the rocket and spinach begin to wilt.*
- *Arrange the stir-fry mixture on plates, top with the salmon fillets, and garnish with fresh flat-leaf parsley and thin strips of fresh red chilli.*

Carbohydrate content per serving: **5** *grams*

Trout

Trout is slightly less rich than salmon, but equally delicious in a different way. Because of its intrinsic flavour, it is, like salmon, simple to cook, the basic aim being to avoid spoiling the natural goodness of the food. Trout can similarly be grilled, poached or baked, but again I prefer baking or poaching to retain the nutrition and texture of the fish.

Trout may be substituted for salmon in all of the previous recipes. It may be served simply with a squeeze of fresh lemon or lime juice, or with lemon butter, lemon and dill butter or lemon and basil butter sauce (see page 103). For some inexplicable reason, the flavour of trout is particularly complemented by nuts – which are an excellent source of vitamin E. It's almost as though nature had planned the gastronomic combination to ensure our continued good health! Trout is usually combined with almonds, which have the dietary advantage of a low carbohydrate content; however, an excellent alternative is pine nuts. The nutritional content is similar and the unique flavours of trout and pine nuts complement one another perfectly. Unlike gastronomic 'experts', I am constrained by the nutritional value and 'dietary potential' of foods. However, in high-quality foods, the dietary potential and nutritional value are virtually identical and effectively equate to the 'taste potential'. Magnificent proteins like fish, meat, poultry and eggs should be enhanced by appropriate natural foods and not overpowered by artificial additives and sauces that detract from the delicious flavours of the foods themselves.

Trout with lemon (or lime) and pine nuts

Trout and pine nuts are a combination made in heaven, both gastronomically and nutritionally. Lemon is not absolutely essential, but it adds a zest that complements the fish, exquisite as this is in splendid isolation! Trout may be grilled in a similar manner to salmon; however, I can see no advantages in this method, either gastronomically or nutritionally. Trout (like most fish) retains nutrients maximally by gentle baking, poaching in a small amount of water, or sautéing in butter with either subtle herb flavours or more simply with lemon or lime juice. What could be simpler, more nutritious or more healthy?

For 2
40 grams butter
2 trout fillets
1 garlic clove, peeled and finely chopped
50 grams pine nuts
juice of a freshly squeezed lemon (or lime)

- *Heat the butter in a shallow frying pan and gently sauté the trout fillets. Add the garlic, pine nuts and the juice of a freshly squeezed lemon (or lime, depending on personal preference). Cook for approximately 3–4 minutes per side (depending on the size of the fish) and serve with a cucumber and mint salad (page 212).*

*Carbohydrate content per serving: **9** grams (including the salad)*

Trout with lemon hollandaise sauce

For 2
200 grams washed fresh spinach
2 large rainbow trout, cleaned
40 grams butter, cubed
freshly ground black pepper
wedges of lemon
sprigs of fresh dill, to garnish

Lemon hollandaise sauce

100 grams butter
1 tbsp white wine vinegar
1 tbsp water
½ bay leaf
4 black peppercorns
2 large free-range egg yolks, separated
1 tbsp freshly squeezed lemon juice
pinch of salt
freshly ground black pepper

- *To prepare the sauce, melt the butter in a medium saucepan and allow to cool. Mix together the white wine vinegar, water, bay leaf and peppercorns in a saucepan, then simmer until the mixture is reduced by half (about 1 tbsp). Sieve, and allow the reduced liquid to cool. Whisk the egg yolks in a heat-safe bowl and beat in the reduced vinegar over simmering water, whisking constantly. When the mixture begins to thicken, slowly add the melted butter, whisking constantly. Add the lemon juice, stirring constantly, season to taste and allow to cool.*
- *Lightly steam the spinach and set aside to cool.*
- *Place the cleaned trout in the base of a shallow oven-proof dish. Dot with the cubes of butter, cover with*

pierced aluminium foil and cook in the centre of a
pre-heated oven at 180 degrees C (gas mark 4) for
20–25 minutes. When cooked, remove the trout from
the dish with a perforated fish-slice and set aside to
cool. Then carefully peel off the skin and place the
trout on a bed of steamed spinach. Season with
freshly ground black pepper, pour the lemon
hollandaise sauce over the trout and serve with a
lemon wedge, garnished with sprigs of fresh dill.

*Carbohydrate content per serving: **1** gram*

Smoked trout pâté

For 2   2 smoked trout fillets
100 grams mascarpone cheese
1 tsp horseradish sauce (page 224)
freshly ground black pepper
half a small red chilli, deseeded and finely chopped
1 tbsp chopped fresh basil
1 tbsp chopped fresh flat-leaf parsley
1 tbsp freshly squeezed lime juice
100 grams clarified butter

- *Flake the fish.*
- *Place the fish in a blender with the mascarpone cheese and horseradish sauce, and blend until smooth.*
- *Add the pepper, chilli, basil, parsley and lime juice and blend again.*
- *Spoon the mixture into ramekin dishes.*
- *Melt the butter in a small saucepan over a gentle heat until it separates.*
- *Pour a little clear butter over the surface of each ramekin.*
- *Cover the ramekins and cool in the fridge.*

Carbohydrate content per serving: **6** *grams*

Lemon sole with pak choi

For 2 4 lemon sole fillets
2 pak choi, halved lengthways
2 tbsp light soy sauce
1 tsp sesame oil
2 tsp fresh coriander, finely chopped
pinch of rock salt
freshly ground black pepper
sprigs of fresh coriander, to garnish

- *Place the lemon sole fillets in a lightly buttered, shallow oven-safe dish, sprinkle with 1 tsp chopped fresh coriander, add sufficient water to just cover the base of the dish, cover and cook in a pre-heated oven at 180 degrees C (gas mark 4) for 12–15 minutes, depending on the size of the fillets.*
- *Whilst the lemon sole fillets are cooking, add water to a large saucepan, to a depth of about 3 cm, bring to the boil, then reduce the heat to a gentle simmer. Lay the pak choi halves in the boiling water, cover and simmer for 2–3 minutes, turning once. Remove the pak choi with a perforated spoon.*
- *Mix together the soy sauce, sesame oil and 1 tsp chopped fresh coriander.*
- *Remove the cooked lemon sole fillets from the baking dish with a fish slice and place on warm plates. Arrange the pak choi halves on the plate and drizzle over the sauce. Garnish with sprigs of fresh coriander.*

Carbohydrate content per serving: negligible

Dover sole with herb sauce

For 2   2 Dover sole
15 grams butter
15 grams plain flour
150 ml full-cream milk
1 tbsp chopped fresh dill
1 tsp chopped fresh chervil
1 tsp chopped fresh flat-leaf parsley
1 tsp freshly squeezed lemon juice
pinch of rock salt
freshly ground black pepper
fresh chervil, to garnish

- *Brush the Dover sole with melted butter and cook under a hot grill for about 8–10 minutes, turning once.*
- *Melt the butter in a small saucepan. Remove from the heat, add the flour and beat to a smooth consistency. Return to a low heat and gradually mix in the milk, constantly stirring to maintain an even consistency. Stir in the chopped dill, chervil, parsley and lemon juice, season to taste and cook for about 2 minutes, stirring constantly.*
- *Serve the sauce over the sole and garnish with fresh chervil.*

*Carbohydrate content per serving: **11** grams*

Tuna with herbs

For 2
4 tbsp extra-virgin olive oil
300 grams fresh tuna, cubed
1 large red onion, peeled and finely sliced
1 garlic clove, peeled and finely chopped
1 medium red pepper, deseeded and chopped
1 medium green pepper, deseeded and chopped
400-gram tin of plum tomatoes, ready-peeled and
   chopped
1 tbsp chopped fresh coriander
1 tbsp chopped fresh basil
1 bay leaf
1 tbsp tomato purée
75 ml dry white wine
pinch of rock salt
freshly ground black pepper
chopped fresh chives, to garnish

- *Heat 3 tablespoons of the olive oil in a large frying pan and brown the tuna on medium heat. Remove the tuna with a perforated spoon, set aside and cover.*
- *Add the remaining tablespoon of olive oil to the pan, stir in the onion, garlic and peppers, and sauté for 1–2 minutes, then add the plum tomatoes (with the juice), herbs, bay leaf, tomato purée and white wine. Simmer for 4–5 minutes, stirring frequently. Return the tuna to the pan, season to taste and simmer for 4–5 minutes. Remove the bay leaf and serve, garnished with chopped fresh chives.*

*Carbohydrate content per serving: **14** grams*

Tuna in dill mayonnaise with mangetout

For 2   200-gram tin of tuna in brine (or springwater), drained
1 tbsp chopped fresh dill
freshly ground black pepper
100 grams French beans
100 grams mangetout
50 grams rocket
Parmesan shavings and fresh dill, to garnish

Mayonnaise

2 free-range egg yolks, separated
1 tbsp freshly squeezed lemon juice
1 tsp Dijon mustard
1 tsp white wine vinegar
250 ml extra-virgin olive oil

- *To prepare mayonnaise, all ingredients must be at room temperature. Blend the egg yolks, lemon juice, mustard and white wine vinegar to a smooth consistency using a whisk or blender. Gradually – and very slowly – add the olive oil whilst stirring, and blend until smooth.*
- *Steam the French beans and mangetout.*
- *Mix 1 tablespoon of the mayonnaise, the tuna and the chopped fresh dill in a bowl and season with freshly ground black pepper. Serve with the French beans and mangetout on a base of rocket and garnish with freshly ground black pepper, shavings of Parmesan cheese and fresh dill.*

*Carbohydrate content per serving: **6** grams*

Tuna with pak choy

For 2   2 tbsp extra-virgin olive oil

2 tuna steaks

3 slices of root ginger, peeled and diced

2 small garlic cloves, peeled and diced

1 medium green chilli, deseeded and finely chopped

juice of a freshly squeezed lemon

2 pak choy, halved

1 tbsp Japanese soy sauce (much lighter than the
    Chinese variety)

- *Heat the extra-virgin olive oil in a medium frying pan
  and gently sear the tuna steaks for approximately
  1 minute, turning once.*
- *Place the tuna steaks on a large sheet of foil.*
- *Top the steaks with the ginger, garlic and chilli.*
- *Drizzle the lemon juice over the tuna.*
- *Place the pak choy around the tuna and then close
  the foil to make a loose parcel.*
- *Place in the centre of a preheated oven at 180
  degrees C (gas mark 4) for about 15 minutes.*
- *Serve immediately.*

Carbohydrate content per serving: **7** *grams*

Cod with basil and chives

For 2   2 cod steak fillets (approximately 150–175 grams each)

1 tbsp chopped fresh chives

25 grams butter, cubed

pinch of rock salt

freshly ground black pepper

3 tbsp extra-virgin olive oil

1 medium onion, peeled and chopped

1 garlic clove, peeled and finely chopped

125 grams button mushrooms, wiped

1 small red pepper, deseeded and sliced

1 small orange pepper, deseeded and sliced

2 medium courgettes, sliced lengthways into quarters

1 tbsp fresh basil, finely chopped

2 tbsp dry sherry

chopped almonds, to garnish

- *Place the cod steaks in the base of a casserole dish, sprinkle over the chives and dot with butter. Season to taste, cover with pierced aluminium foil and bake in the centre of a pre-heated oven at 180 degrees C (gas mark 4) for 12–15 minutes.*
- *Heat the olive oil in a wok and sauté the onion and garlic for about a minute, then add the mushrooms, peppers, courgettes, basil and sherry. Cook for 2–3 minutes, stirring frequently.*
- *Serve the sauce over the cod steaks and garnish with chopped almonds.*

*Carbohydrate content per serving: **11** grams*

Cod with tomato and coriander salsa

For 2   2 cod steaks, approximately 150 grams each
1 tbsp extra-virgin olive oil
tomato and coriander salsa (see page 206)
pinch of rock salt
freshly ground black pepper
fresh coriander leaves, to garnish

- *Brush the cod steaks with the olive oil and grill on a high heat for 6–7 minutes, turning once. Season to taste and serve on warm plates with the tomato and coriander salsa, garnished with fresh coriander.*

*Carbohydrate content per serving: **7** grams*

Cod with parsley sauce
A classic recipe – which is also perfect for a low-carbohydrate diet.

For 2   2 cod steaks, approximately 150 grams each
15 grams unsalted butter
15 grams plain flour
150 ml full-cream milk
1 tbsp chopped fresh flat-leaf parsley
freshly ground black pepper
150 grams baby leeks
fresh flat-leaf parsley, to garnish

- *Place the cod steaks in the base of a buttered, shallow, oven-safe dish, add sufficient water to just cover the base of the dish, cover and bake in the centre of a pre-heated oven at 180 degrees C (gas mark 4) for 12–14 minutes. Remove from the oven and place the cod steaks on warm plates.*
- *While the cod is baking, heat the butter in a small saucepan, then remove from the heat and gradually stir in the flour. Return to a low heat and gradually add the milk, stirring constantly. When the mixture reaches an even consistency and is just beginning to thicken, remove from the heat and mix in the parsley. Season with freshly ground black pepper and pour over the cod steaks.*
- *Lightly steam the baby leeks and serve with the cod. Garnish with fresh flat-leaf parsley.*

*Carbohydrate content per serving: **12** grams*

Mackerel

Mackerel is a very rich fish, high in essential omega-3 fatty acids and vitamin D. It is an acquired taste, and people seem to either love it or loathe it. If you haven't tried mackerel, please do. For some reason, which I have never understood, it is not one of the most popular fish, but it is certainly one of the most tasty and nutritious.

Smoked mackerel pâté

For 2
1 smoked mackerel fillet
2 tbsp soured cream
50 grams Philadelphia cream cheese
1 tbsp chopped fresh chives
1 tsp freshly squeezed lemon juice
pinch of rock salt
freshly ground black pepper
pinch of cayenne pepper and some lemon zest, to
    garnish

- *Flake the smoked mackerel to remove all bones and skin. Put it in a blender with the soured cream, cream cheese, chopped chives and lemon juice. Season to taste, and purée until smooth. Transfer to a medium bowl and chill for 2–3 hours before serving.*
- *Serve the smoked mackerel pâté with a crispy green salad (see page 209), garnished with a pinch of cayenne pepper and some lemon zest.*

*Carbohydrate content per serving: **5** grams (including salad)*

Mackerel with lemon and coriander

For 2   2 mackerel fillets
juice of a freshly squeezed lemon
1 tbsp chopped fresh coriander
25 grams unsalted butter, cubed
lemon wedges
½ tbsp fresh coriander leaves, to garnish

- *Place the mackerel fillets in the base of a shallow, oven-safe casserole dish, squeeze over them the juice of half a lemon and sprinkle on the chopped fresh coriander. Arrange the butter cubes evenly over the mackerel, then cover with pierced aluminium foil and cook in the centre of a pre-heated oven at 180 degrees C (gas mark 4) for 15–18 minutes. Serve with lemon wedges, garnish with fresh coriander leaves and serve with a salad.*

Carbohydrate content per serving: 3 grams

Smoked mackerel with crushed black pepper
Smoked mackerel is such a rich dish, full of natural flavours, that it requires very little accompaniment. Crushed black peppercorns complement the richness of the mackerel perfectly.

For 2
2 smoked mackerel fillets
8–10 black peppercorns, crushed
2 tbsp extra-virgin olive oil
100 grams French beans
sprigs of fresh dill, to garnish

- *Brush the mackerel fillets on both sides with extra-virgin olive oil and coat the fillets with the crushed peppercorns. Place under a hot grill and cook for 3–4 minutes per side, turning once.*
- *Serve with lightly steamed French beans and garnish with sprigs of fresh dill.*

Carbohydrate content per serving: **3** *grams*

Mackerel with honey and orange

For 2   2 mackerel, 150 grams each, cleaned and heads
         removed

Marinade

         2 tbsp extra-virgin olive oil
         2 tbsp freshly squeezed lime juice
         2 tbsp freshly squeezed orange juice
         1 tbsp runny honey
         freshly ground black pepper

- *Make 4 diagonal slashes along both sides of the mackerel.*
- *Mix together the marinade and marinate the mackerel for approximately 1 hour.*
- *Place the mackerel under a moderate grill (no closer than 8 cm) for approximately 4–5 minutes per side, turning once.*
- *Serve immediately with a crispy green salad (page 209).*

*Carbohydrate content per serving: **10** grams*

Whiting with ginger and lime

For 2
2 tbsp extra-virgin olive oil
2 shallots, peeled and finely diced
1 garlic clove, peeled and finely chopped
4 whiting fillets, approximately 75–80 grams each
75 grams butter
2 tsp freshly squeezed lime juice
½ tsp freshly grated lime rind
2 slices fresh ginger, peeled and grated
1 tbsp chopped fresh dill
pinch of rock salt
freshly ground black pepper
lime wedges
sprigs of fresh dill, to garnish
150 grams sugar snap peas
100 grams button mushrooms, wiped and halved

- *Heat the olive oil in a large frying pan and sauté the diced shallots and garlic.*
- *Lightly sauté the whiting fillets, turning once.*
- *Melt the butter in a small saucepan; stir in the lime juice, lime rind and fresh ginger, and gently heat for 1–2 minutes. Add the chopped dill and season to taste. Transfer the whiting fillets to warm plates, spoon the sauce over the fillets and garnish with sprigs of fresh dill and lime wedges.*
- *Steam the sugar snap peas and sauté the mushrooms in butter. Serve with the whiting.*

Carbohydrate content per serving: 7 grams

Haddock with peppers and ginger

For 2   2 tbsp extra-virgin olive oil
1 red onion, peeled and diced
1 garlic clove, peeled and finely chopped
2 slices fresh root ginger, peeled and finely chopped
1 small red pepper, deseeded and finely sliced
1 small green pepper, deseeded and finely sliced
1 small yellow pepper, deseeded and finely sliced
1 tbsp chopped fresh dill
1 tbsp chopped fresh chervil
pinch of rock salt
freshly ground black pepper
2 large haddock fillets, approximately 150 grams each
25 grams butter, melted
1 tbsp chopped fresh chives, to garnish

- *Heat the olive oil in a wok and sauté the onion and garlic for about a minute. Add the ginger, peppers, chervil and dill, and season to taste. Stir-fry for 2–3 minutes, stirring frequently.*
- *Spoon the vegetables on to two large aluminium foil rectangles, lay the haddock fillets on the bed of vegetables, brush with melted butter and season with freshly ground black pepper. Close the aluminium parcels loosely, then cook in the centre of a pre-heated oven at 180 degrees C (gas mark 4) for about 15 minutes. Serve in the opened parcels, garnished with chopped fresh chives.*

*Carbohydrate content per serving: **10** grams*

Chilli and lime swordfish

For 2 2 tbsp extra-virgin olive oil
1 green chilli, deseeded and chopped finely
juice of 2 freshly squeezed limes
1 tbsp chopped fresh coriander leaves
1 tbsp chopped fresh basil leaves
2 swordfish steaks, approximately 150 grams each

- *Mix together the olive oil, chilli, lime juice, coriander and basil in a large bowl.*
- *Coat the swordfish steaks with the mixture.*
- *Place the swordfish steaks in a medium roasting tin and cover with pierced aluminium foil.*
- *Cook in the centre of a preheated oven at 180 degrees C (gas mark 4) for approximately 20 minutes.*
- *Serve immediately with a crispy green salad (page 209).*

*Carbohydrate content per serving: **4 grams***

Monkfish with sweet and sour peppers

For 2
1 green pepper, deseeded and sliced
1 red pepper, deseeded and sliced
1 red onion, peeled and sliced
2 tsp granulated sugar
1 tbsp white wine vinegar
2 monkfish fillets
butter
freshly ground black pepper
fresh coriander leaves, to garnish

- *Place the peppers and onion in an ovenproof dish. Sprinkle with sugar and drizzle over the white wine vinegar. Cover with perforated aluminium foil and cook in a preheated oven at 180 degrees C (gas mark 4) for about 25–30 minutes.*
- *Place the monkfish in a separate roasting dish. Dot with butter, cover with perforated aluminium foil and cook for approximately 20 minutes.*
- *Place the monkfish fillets on plates, and top with the sweet and sour peppers. Season to taste and garnish with fresh coriander leaves.*

*Carbohydrate content per serving: **12** grams*

Monkfish with herbs

For 2   2 tbsp extra-virgin olive oil
2 medium monkfish fillets, approximately 150 grams
   each
2 shallots, peeled and sliced
1 garlic clove, peeled and finely chopped
300 grams white button mushrooms, halved
   lengthways
1 tbsp chopped fresh basil leaves
1 tbsp chopped fresh flat-leaf parsley

- *Heat 1 tablespoon of extra-virgin olive oil in a medium frying pan and cook the monkfish for approximately 8 minutes, turning once.*
- *Remove from the pan and set aside.*
- *Add the remaining extra-virgin olive oil to the pan and sauté the shallots and garlic for about 2 minutes.*
- *Add the mushrooms, basil and flat-leaf parsley and stir-fry for about 4–5 minutes.*
- *Serve the fish immediately, topped with the mushroom and herb mixture.*

*Carbohydrate content per serving: **10** grams*

Bream teriyaki

For 2   2 tbsp saki
2 tbsp Japanese soy sauce
2 slices of fresh ginger, peeled and finely chopped
1 garlic clove, peeled and finely chopped
2 sea bream fillets, skin on
3 tbsp extra-virgin olive oil
a few drops of linseed oil
100 grams kale
100 grams bean sprouts
2 spring onions, trimmed and chopped diagonally into
    2-cm segments
freshly ground black pepper

- *Mix together the saki, soy sauce, ginger, garlic and linseed oil and marinate the bream for approximately 1 hour in the fridge.*
- *Heat the extra-virgin olive oil in a frying pan and cook the bream, skin side down, for approximately 3 minutes.*
- *Pour the marinade over the bream, turn the fish and cook for a further 3–4 minutes.*

At the same time
- *Heat 1 tbsp extra-virgin olive oil in a wok and stir-fry the kale, bean sprouts and spring onions for 3–4 minutes.*
- *Arrange the stir-fried vegetables on a plate topped with the sea bream, and season with black pepper to taste.*
- *Serve immediately.*

*Carbohydrate content per serving: **6** grams*

Chapter 10 Shellfish

Shellfish are an individual taste: people seem either to love or loathe shellfish, but there can be no denying their superb nutritional value.

Incidentally, you will notice that 'tiger prawns' can include a variety of different species of different sizes, from Crevettes (at 6–8 cm) to larger specimens up to 15 cm, depending on the fishmonger. In the following recipes, tiger prawns are the 6–8-cm variety.

Chilli tiger prawns with mangetout

For 2
2 tbsp extra-virgin olive oil
1 garlic clove, peeled and finely chopped
2 spring onions, chopped into 4–5-cm lengths
100 grams mangetout
1 small green chilli, deseeded and finely chopped
250 grams cooked tiger prawns, peeled and deveined
1 tbsp sweet sherry
pinch of rock salt
freshly ground black pepper
sesame oil
chopped fresh chives, to garnish

- *Heat the olive oil and sauté the garlic, spring onions, mangetout and chilli for about 2 minutes. Add the cooked tiger prawns and sherry. Season to taste and stir-fry for another 2 minutes, stirring frequently. Serve on warm plates, drizzle over a few drops of sesame oil and garnish with chopped fresh chives.*

Carbohydrate content per serving: 6 grams

Tiger prawn salad with avocado lime dressing

For 2   300 grams cooked tiger prawns, shelled and
          deveined
          1 tbsp freshly squeezed lime juice
          3 tbsp dry white wine
          100 grams mixed curly green lettuce leaves (curly
          endive, mizuna, cos and green coral)
          2 spring onions, chopped into 4–5 cm lengths
          lime zest, to garnish

Dressing

          1 small ripe Hass avocado, halved, stoned and diced
          2 shallots, peeled and chopped
          1 tbsp freshly squeezed lime juice
          2 tbsp extra-virgin olive oil
          freshly ground black pepper

- *Marinate the cooked tiger prawns, lime juice and white wine for 2–3 hours in the fridge.*
- *Blend the avocado, shallots, lime juice, olive oil and freshly ground black pepper (either with a blender or by hand) until smooth.*
- *Mix the lettuce leaves and spring onions in a large salad bowl, arrange the tiger prawns on the lettuce and spoon the avocado dressing on the salad. Garnish with lime zest.*

*Carbohydrate content per serving: **4** grams*

Tiger prawns with basil and tomatoes

For 2
2 tsp sesame seeds
2 tbsp extra-virgin olive oil
3 spring onions, peeled and chopped into 4–5-cm
   lengths
1 garlic clove, peeled and finely chopped
1 small red pepper, deseeded and finely sliced
200-gram tin of plum tomatoes, chopped
2 tsp tomato purée
1 tbsp sweet sherry
pinch of rock salt
freshly ground black pepper
250 grams cooked tiger prawns, shelled and
   deveined
1 tbsp fresh basil, finely chopped
sprigs of fresh oregano, to garnish

- *Lightly toast the sesame seeds and set aside.*
- *Heat the olive oil in the wok until hot, add the spring onions and garlic, and sauté for 1–2 minutes. Add the sliced red pepper and cook for a further minute, stirring frequently, then add the tomatoes, tomato purée and sherry, and season to taste. Simmer for 1–2 minutes. Finally, add the pre-cooked tiger prawns and chopped basil, and simmer gently for a further 4–5 minutes. Serve immediately, garnished with fresh oregano and sesame seeds.*

Carbohydrate content per serving: **9** *grams*

Prawns with rocket salad

For 2   3 tbsp extra-virgin olive oil
250 grams cooked prawns
handful of rocket leaves
1 small ripe Hass avocado, halved, stoned, peeled
   and finely sliced
freshly ground black pepper
1 tbsp chopped chives
lime wedges

Sauce

100 grams unsalted butter
2 tsp freshly squeezed lemon juice
freshly ground black pepper
1 tbsp chopped fresh chives
1 tbsp chopped fresh chervil
1 tbsp chopped fresh basil

- *Melt the butter in a small saucepan and stir in the lemon juice, freshly ground black pepper, chives, chervil and basil.*
- *Heat the olive oil in a saucepan and sauté the prawns for 2–3 minutes. Remove from the pan and cover.*
- *Arrange the avocado slices like the spokes of a wheel, centred in the middle of the plate. Place the rocket leaves on the avocado and season with freshly ground black pepper. Place the cooked prawns on the rocket and pour the herb butter sauce over them. Serve with lime wedges and garnish with chopped chives.*

*Carbohydrate content per serving: **2** grams*

Prawns in garlic butter
Easy and quick to prepare, this recipe tastes delicious and is nutritionally superb, with virtually no carbohydrate content. Simply perfect!

For 2   300 grams raw tiger prawns, shelled
3 tbsp extra-virgin olive oil
2 garlic cloves, peeled and finely chopped
chopped fresh coriander, to garnish

- *The easiest way to shell a prawn is to break off the head and tail, remove the legs, and the shell will then peel off easily and quickly. Using a sharp knife – and great care – slice down the back of the prawn and devein (remove the dark thread) by washing under running water.*
- *Heat the extra-virgin olive oil and sauté the garlic for approximately 30–40 seconds. Add the peeled prawns and cook – stirring regularly – for 3–4 minutes, depending upon the size of the prawns, until cooked. Remove the prawns from the pan and cover.*
- *Prepare a garlic butter sauce according to the recipe on page 145, pour over the prawns and garnish with chopped fresh coriander.*

Carbohydrate content per serving: negligible

Scallops with lime and ginger

For 2   250 grams fresh scallops, cleaned
3 tbsp extra-virgin olive oil
100 grams mangetout
3 shallots, peeled and quartered
1 garlic clove, peeled and grated
2 slices of fresh ginger root, peeled and finely
    chopped
1 small red pepper, deseeded and finely sliced
75 grams button mushrooms, wiped and halved
freshly ground black pepper
lime wedges
fresh tarragon, to garnish

Marinade
2 tbsp light soy sauce
1 tbsp sweet sherry
1 slice fresh ginger root, peeled and finely chopped
1 garlic clove, peeled and grated
1 tbsp freshly squeezed lime juice
1 tsp cornflour

- *Mix together the ingredients of the marinade, add the scallops and marinate in the fridge for 2–3 hours.*
- *Heat 2 tablespoons of the olive oil in a wok, add the scallops and sauté gently for about 3 minutes. Remove the scallops with a perforated spoon, set aside and cover. Heat the remaining olive oil in the wok, add the mangetout, shallots, garlic, ginger and red pepper, and cook for 2 minutes, stirring frequently. Return the scallops to the wok, add the mushrooms, and season with freshly ground black pepper. Cook on medium heat for another 3 minutes and serve with wedges of lime, garnished with fresh tarragon.*

*Carbohydrate content per serving: **12** grams*

Scallops and asparagus with sweet chilli sauce
Scallops and asparagus complement one another wonderfully in every respect: taste, texture and nutritional content. This recipe has extra zest – and vitamins – when fresh chilli is included; however, it is still delicious and nutritious without chilli, for those who prefer life less hot!

For 2
- 1 bunch of fresh asparagus, trimmed and chopped into 5–6-cm lengths
- 3 tbsp extra-virgin olive oil
- 1 garlic clove, peeled and finely chopped
- 2 shallots, finely chopped
- 250 grams cleaned, fresh scallops
- 1 small red chilli, deseeded and finely chopped (optional)
- 2 tbsp light soy sauce
- 2 tbsp sweet sherry
- ½ tsp granulated sugar
- 30 grams melted butter
- freshly ground black pepper
- fresh coriander leaves, to garnish

- *Lightly steam the asparagus, transfer to a warm plate and cover.*
- *Heat the extra-virgin olive oil in the wok and sauté the garlic, shallots, scallops and chilli over medium heat for 3–4 minutes. Add the soy sauce, sherry, sugar and melted butter, season with freshly ground black pepper, and cook for a further 2 minutes. Arrange the asparagus aesthetically on warm plates, serve the chilli scallops on the asparagus and garnish with fresh coriander leaves.*

Carbohydrate content per serving: **4** *grams*

Ginger scallops with mangetout

For 2   3 tbsp extra-virgin olive oil
250 grams fresh, cleaned scallops
1 garlic clove, peeled and finely chopped
3 slices of fresh ginger root, peeled and finely chopped
100 grams mangetout
1 small red pepper, deseeded and finely sliced
1 tbsp light soy sauce
2 tbsp freshly squeezed orange juice
freshly ground black pepper
chopped fresh chives, to garnish

* *Heat the extra-virgin olive oil in the wok, add the scallops and sauté for 2–3 minutes. Remove the scallops carefully (to prevent breaking) with a perforated spoon. Add the garlic and ginger to the wok, and stir-fry for 30–40 seconds, then add the mangetout and pepper, and sauté for a further 2 minutes. Return the scallops to the wok, add the soy sauce and orange juice, stir gently and cook for a final 2–3 minutes. Serve garnished with chopped fresh chives.*

Carbohydrate content per serving: **7** *grams*

Mussels in garlic sauce

For 2   750 grams fresh mussels, bearded and scrubbed
2 tbsp fresh thyme, finely chopped
1 medium onion, peeled and diced
pinch of rock salt
freshly ground black pepper
150 ml dry white wine
100 grams butter
4 garlic cloves, peeled and grated
sprigs of fresh thyme, to garnish

- *Wash and scrub the mussels several times, discarding any that are open. When you are completely satisfied regarding the safety of the mussels, place them in a large saucepan with the chopped thyme, onion, salt, freshly ground black pepper and wine.*
- *Bring to the boil, then cover and simmer on a high heat until the mussels open (usually 5–7 minutes); remember only to use those which have opened.*
- *Remove the opened mussels with a perforated spoon and transfer to a shallow casserole dish. Cover and place in the centre of a warm oven.*
- *Strain the mixture, return the remaining liquid to the pan and reduce by about half. Add the butter and finely grated garlic, simmer gently for 2–3 minutes and pour over the mussels. Garnish with sprigs of fresh thyme.*

*Carbohydrate content per serving: **4** grams*

Mussels with coriander

For 2   750 grams fresh mussels, bearded and scrubbed
150 ml dry white wine
2 shallots, peeled and finely chopped
freshly ground black pepper
2 garlic cloves, peeled and finely chopped
4 tbsp chopped fresh coriander leaves
extra virgin-olive oil
flat-leaf parsley, to garnish

- *Wash and scrub the mussels several times, discarding any that are open.*
- *Place the mussels in a large saucepan with the garlic, wine, shallots and freshly ground black pepper, bring to the boil and simmer on a high heat until the mussels open (approximately 6–7 minutes).*
- *Only use mussels that are open. Unopened mussels should be discarded.*
- *Remove the open mussels with a perforated spoon and transfer to a shallow casserole dish.*
- *Cover and place in the centre of a warm oven.*
- *Strain the mixture and reduce the liquid in the pan by about half.*
- *Simmer gently with the coriander for 1–2 minutes and pour over the mussels.*
- *Drizzle with some extra-virgin olive oil and garnish with some sprigs of flat-leaf parsley.*

Carbohydrate content per serving: **5** *grams*

Prawn soufflé

For 2   2 tbsp extra-virgin olive oil
1 garlic clove, peeled and finely chopped
1 green chilli, deseeded and finely chopped
35 grams cooked prawns, shelled and deveined
4 free-range eggs, separated
25 grams butter
25 grams plain flour
150 ml full-cream milk
1 tbsp chopped fresh basil leaves
freshly ground black pepper
fresh parsley leaves, to garnish

- *In a medium saucepan, heat the extra-virgin olive oil and sauté the garlic and chilli for 1–2 minutes.*
- *Stir in the prawns and cook over a medium heat for 2 minutes.*
- *Separate the eggs, beat the yolks, and whisk the whites until firm.*
- *Melt the butter in a small saucepan and then gradually beat in the flour and milk until the mixture has thickened.*
- *Remove from the heat and allow to stand for 2–3 minutes, stirring occasionally.*
- *Fold in the egg yolks, stir in the flour mixture and basil and season to taste.*
- *Stir in the sautéed prawns, garlic and chilli.*
- *Beat a tablespoon of egg white into the mixture.*
- *Spoon the mixture evenly into a buttered soufflé dish.*
- *Bake in the centre of preheated oven at 180 degrees C (gas mark 4) for 30–35 minutes.*
- *Serve immediately, garnished with parsley.*

*Carbohydrate content per serving: **12** grams*

Calamari with mixed pepper salsa

For 2   3 tbsp extra-virgin olive oil
         500 grams calamari rings
         100 grams wild rocket leaves
         freshly ground black pepper

Salsa

         1 small red pepper, deseeded and diced
         1 small yellow pepper, deseeded and diced
         1 small green chilli, deseeded and diced
         1 tbsp finely chopped fresh basil leaves
         1 tbsp finely chopped fresh coriander leaves

- Heat the extra-virgin olive oil in a wok and stir-fry the calamari for 2–3 minutes.
- Mix together the peppers, chilli, basil and coriander in a small bowl.
- Arrange a bed of wild rocket on the plates, and top with the calamari rings.
- Spoon the salsa over the squid and season to taste with freshly ground black pepper.

Carbohydrate content per serving: **6** *grams*

Chapter 11 Meat

It is very important in a diet of this nature to include foods cooked in the most natural manner, because these foods have natural flavours and nutrition which simply cannot be reproduced by artificial procedures. And whilst we can – and will – add nutritious sauces and accompaniments, it is essential to bear in mind that the meat (or fish, or poultry, or shellfish) is the real star of the meal; the sauces will (hopefully) enhance, but merely play the supporting role.

Grilled pepper steak with French beans

For 2   2 sirloin or fillet steaks, about 150 grams each, and no
more than 2.5 cm thick
2 tbsp extra-virgin olive oil
freshly ground black pepper
100 grams French beans

- *Brush the steaks with olive oil on both sides and season liberally with freshly ground black pepper. Place under a hot grill, at least 8 cm from the source of heat, and grill to taste, turning once.*
- *Steam the French beans until tender but still firm. The French beans can be simply served with the steaks or with one of the sauces below.*

Carbohydrate content per serving: negligible

....

Lemon butter sauce

60 grams unsalted butter
juice of ½ a freshly squeezed lemon
freshly ground black pepper

- *Heat the butter in a small saucepan, stir in the lemon juice and freshly ground pepper, to taste, and serve.*

*Carbohydrate content per serving: **2** grams*

Garlic butter sauce

75 grams unsalted butter
2 garlic cloves, peeled and grated
1 tsp chopped flat-leaf parsley
1 tsp lemon juice
freshly ground black pepper

- *Heat the butter in a small saucepan, stir in the garlic, parsley, lemon juice and freshly ground black pepper, and serve.*

*Carbohydrate content per serving: **2** grams*

Ginger and oyster sauce

1 tbsp extra-virgin olive oil
2–3 drops sesame oil
1 garlic clove, peeled and finely chopped
1 tsp oyster sauce
2 slices of fresh ginger root, peeled and finely chopped
1 tbsp sweet sherry
2 tbsp water
freshly ground black pepper

- *Heat the olive oil and sesame oil in a small saucepan, add the garlic and sauté for about a minute. Add the oyster sauce, ginger root, sherry and water and cook on medium heat for approximately 2 minutes, stirring frequently. Serve.*

*Carbohydrate content per serving: **4** grams*

Beef casserole with chives

Tinned tomatoes are deliberately utilised in this dish, as they seem to provide an even richer source of lycopene (that marvellous antioxidant) than do fresh tomatoes.

Beef casserole can be served with numerous accompaniments; try lightly steamed broccoli florets, fresh peas, French beans or mangetout; the average serving only adds about 2–4 grams of carbohydrate to the meal.

For 2   400 grams casserole steak, chopped into large
              cubes
          pinch of rock salt
          2 tsp dry English mustard
          freshly ground black pepper
          1 tbsp plain flour
          50 grams butter
          2 large onions, peeled and chopped
          1 large garlic clove, peeled and finely chopped
          1 large carrot, peeled and sliced
          400-gram tin of plum tomatoes, ready-peeled
          200 ml beef stock
          2 tbsp chopped fresh chives

- *Coat the meat with flour, then mix it with the salt, dry mustard and freshly ground pepper in a large bowl.*
- *Heat the butter and sauté the onions and garlic for approximately 1–2 minutes, or until soft. Add the meat and brown for 2–3 minutes. Then gradually blend in the carrot, tomatoes (including the juice) and stock, and season to taste. Spoon into a casserole dish, cover and cook for about 2 hours at 180 degrees C (gas mark 4). Serve topped with freshly chopped chives.*

*Carbohydrate content per serving: **21** grams*

Moussaka

For 2
1 large fresh aubergine, sliced
pinch of rock salt
3 tbsp extra-virgin olive oil
1 large onion, peeled and finely chopped
1 medium garlic clove, peeled and finely chopped
250 grams beef mince
3 large plum tomatoes, peeled and chopped
1 tbsp tomato purée
75 ml beef stock
freshly ground black pepper

Sauce

15 grams butter
15 grams plain flour
150 ml full-cream milk
50 grams grated cheese (preferably, but not
    essentially, Greek Kefalotyri)
freshly ground black pepper

- *Clean and slice the aubergine, then arrange in salted layers in a colander for 30 minutes. Rinse thoroughly and pat dry. Arrange the aubergine slices in a single layer on a baking tray, brush with a thin layer of olive oil and cook in a pre-heated oven at 180 degrees C (gas mark 4) for 10 minutes. Remove from the oven and set aside to cool.*
- *Heat 2 tablespoons of the olive oil and sauté the onion and garlic for 1–2 minutes until soft, then add the minced beef, stirring regularly until evenly browned. Add the chopped tomatoes and tomato purée, and stir in the stock. Season to taste and gently simmer for 10–15 minutes.*

- *Arrange half the aubergine slices in the base of an oven-proof casserole dish, add the beef mixture, then top with a second layer of aubergine slices.*
- *To prepare the sauce, heat the butter in a saucepan until melted, remove from the heat and gradually mix in the flour, stirring constantly. Return to a low heat and slowly add the milk, stirring constantly. When the mixture has reached an even consistency, add the grated cheese and stir until evenly melted into the sauce. Season to taste.*
- *Pour the sauce over the mixture in the casserole dish, top with a little grated cheese and bake in a pre-heated oven for 35–40 minutes at 180 degrees C (gas mark 4).*
- *Serve with Feta salad (see page 205).*

*Carbohydrate content per serving: **27** grams (including salad)*

Beef stroganoff

For 2 4 tbsp extra-virgin olive oil
1 large onion, peeled and finely sliced
1 garlic clove, peeled and finely chopped
75 grams button mushrooms, wiped and halved
1 tbsp plain flour
pinch of rock salt
freshly ground black pepper
250 grams fillet steak, sliced in thin strips
1 tsp tomato purée
100 ml beef stock
1 tbsp chopped fresh basil
1 tbsp chopped fresh parsley
100 ml soured cream
1 tbsp chopped fresh chives, to garnish

- *Heat 2 tablespoons of the extra-virgin olive oil in a large pan and sauté the onion and garlic for approximately 1 minute. Add the mushrooms and sauté for a further minute. Transfer to a casserole dish, cover and place in a warm oven, 140 degrees C (gas mark 1).*
- *Coat the steak in seasoned flour.*
- *Heat the remaining olive oil in the pan and brown the steak, stirring regularly. Return the onion, garlic and mushrooms to the pan, and add the stock, tomato purée and fresh herbs. Simmer for 12–15 minutes, remove from the heat and stir in the soured cream. Serve immediately, garnished with chopped fresh chives.*

*Carbohydrate content per serving: **12** grams*

Sliced beef in oyster sauce

For 2   250 grams steak, sliced into thin strips
           3 tbsp extra-virgin olive oil
           1 garlic clove, peeled and finely chopped
           2 slices of fresh ginger root, peeled and finely
               chopped
           100 grams mushrooms, wiped and halved (the dish
               will have a better aesthetic appearance if you use
               a mixture of different mushrooms, but the
               nutritional value is the same for all mushrooms)
           4 spring onions, chopped into 3–4-cm lengths
           100 grams broccoli florets
           1 small red pepper, deseeded and finely sliced
           ½ tsp granulated sugar
           freshly ground black pepper
           1 green chilli, deseeded and cut into strips, to garnish
               (optional)

Marinade

           1 tbsp light soy sauce
           1 tbsp oyster sauce
           1 tbsp sweet sherry
           1 tsp cornflour

- *Mix the soy sauce, oyster sauce, sherry and cornflour
  to an even consistency, then add to the sliced beef in
  a large bowl. Marinate in the fridge for 3–4 hours.*
- *Heat 2 tablespoons of the extra-virgin olive oil in the
  wok and stir-fry the beef for 2 minutes. Add the
  ginger and garlic and cook for a further 2 minutes,
  stirring constantly. Remove from the wok with a
  perforated spoon and set aside.*

- *Heat the remaining olive oil in the wok, add the mushrooms, broccoli, spring onions and red pepper, and stir-fry for 2–3 minutes. Return the beef to the wok, add the oyster sauce marinade and sugar, and stir-fry for a further 2–3 minutes. Season with freshly ground black pepper and serve garnished with green chilli strips.*

Carbohydrate content per serving: 16 grams

Steak and asparagus

For 2   2 sirloin or fillet steaks, about 150 grams each, and no
more than 2.5 cm thick
1 tbsp extra-virgin olive oil
freshly ground black pepper
200 grams fresh asparagus

- *Brush the steaks with olive oil, season with freshly ground black pepper and grill to taste, turning once.*
- *Lightly steam the asparagus until tender but firm. Serve with one of the following sauces.*

Carbohydrate content per serving: negligible

Lemon butter sauce
(See page 144.)

*Carbohydrate content per serving: **2** grams*

Herb butter sauce

75 grams unsalted butter
1 tsp chopped fresh chives
1 tsp chopped fresh rosemary
pinch of paprika
1 tsp freshly squeezed lemon juice
freshly ground black pepper

- *Melt the butter in a small saucepan, then stir in the chives, rosemary, paprika and lemon juice. Season with freshly ground black pepper and serve over the asparagus.*

*Carbohydrate content per serving: **2** grams*

Pot-roast beef

For 4
1 kilogram rolled brisket of beef
4 tbsp extra-virgin olive oil
2 medium onions, peeled and chopped
1 garlic clove, peeled and finely chopped
1 tbsp plain flour
500 ml beef stock
200 grams carrots, peeled and sliced on the diagonal
100 grams swede, peeled and cubed
1 bay leaf
1 tbsp fresh flat-leaf parsley, finely chopped
2 tsp tomato purée
1 tsp dry mustard
pinch of rock salt
freshly ground black pepper
sprigs of fresh flat-leaf parsley, to garnish

- *Heat the olive oil in a large saucepan and brown the brisket of beef thoroughly on all sides. Remove the beef from the pan (leaving the juices in the pan), place in a large casserole dish and cover.*
- *Add the onions and garlic to the pan and sauté for 1–2 minutes. Stir in the flour, then gradually stir in the stock. Add the remainder of the vegetables and simmer for a further 3–4 minutes. Stir in the bay leaf, parsley, tomato purée and mustard. Season to taste, then add to the casserole dish, mixing well. Cover and place in the centre of a pre-heated oven at 140 degrees C (gas mark 1) for about 2 hours.*
- *Test the meat to ensure that it is tender. Remove the bay leaf and garnish with fresh flat-leaf parsley.*

Carbohydrate content per serving: **17** grams

Goulash

For 2   2 tbsp plain flour
1 tbsp paprika
pinch of rock salt
freshly ground black pepper
250 grams casserole steak, chopped into 4–5-cm cubes
2 tbsp extra-virgin olive oil
1 large onion, peeled and chopped
1 garlic clove, peeled and finely chopped
200-gram tin of plum tomatoes, chopped
2 tsp tomato purée
150 ml beef stock
2 tsp chopped fresh dill
2 tsp chopped fresh thyme
2 tsp chopped fresh parsley
100 ml soured cream
sprigs of fresh thyme, to garnish

- *Mix the flour with the paprika and season with salt and freshly ground black pepper. Coat the steak in the seasoned flour. Heat 2 tbsp of olive oil in a frying pan and brown the steak. Add the onion and garlic and sauté for about 1 minute. Add the tomatoes, tomato purée, stock and herbs, stirring constantly. Season to taste and simmer for about an hour. Stir in the soured cream and serve immediately, garnished with sprigs of fresh thyme.*

Carbohydrate content per serving: **21** grams

Beef kebabs

For 2   250 grams lean steak, cubed

1 large red pepper, deseeded and chopped into 3-cm cubes

12 button mushrooms, wiped and trimmed

1 large green pepper, deseeded and chopped into 3-cm cubes

12 baby yellow squash

freshly ground black pepper

3 tbsp extra-virgin olive oil

2 tbsp chopped fresh chives, to garnish

Marinade

2 tbsp dry sherry

1 tbsp light soy sauce

1 garlic clove, peeled and finely chopped

1 slice of fresh ginger root, peeled and finely chopped

1 tsp freshly squeezed lemon juice

1 tsp honey

pinch of rock salt

freshly ground black pepper

- *Marinate the steak for 2–3 hours. Soak the wooden skewers in water for a similar period.*
- *Thread the steak, peppers, button mushrooms and squash on the skewers. Brush with extra-virgin olive oil and season with freshly ground black pepper, then grill (or barbecue) until the meat is cooked to taste. Garnish with chopped fresh chives, and serve with a cucumber and bean sprout salad (see page 211).*

*Carbohydrate content per serving: **11** grams (including salad)*

Cabernet Sauvignon beef

For 2   300 grams casserole steak, chopped into 4–5-cm cubes
2 tbsp plain flour
pinch of rock salt
freshly ground black pepper
3 tbsp extra-virgin olive oil
300 ml Cabernet Sauvignon red wine
1 garlic clove, peeled and finely chopped
1 bay leaf
1 tsp tomato purée
1 tbsp chopped fresh thyme
1 tbsp chopped fresh sage
25 grams butter
8 baby onions, peeled
100 grams button mushrooms, wiped and halved
75 grams carrots, julienned
75 grams French beans
75 grams broccoli florets

- *Coat the steak in seasoned flour, heat the olive oil in a large frying pan and brown the steak. Slowly add the Cabernet Sauvignon, and stir in the garlic, bay leaf, tomato purée, thyme and sage. Season to taste and transfer to an oven-safe casserole dish.*
- *In a separate pan, melt the butter and sauté the onions and mushrooms lightly. Transfer the onions and mushrooms to the casserole dish and stir gently. Cover, and cook in the centre of a pre-heated oven for 2 hours at 140 degrees C (gas mark 1).*
- *Serve with lightly steamed carrots, French beans and broccoli florets.*

Carbohydrate content per serving: **22** *grams*

Sweet and sour pork

For 2   2 tbsp plain flour
pinch of rock salt
freshly ground black pepper
250 grams lean pork fillet, sliced thinly on the diagonal
3 tbsp extra-virgin olive oil
4 spring onions, chopped into 4–5-cm lengths
1 garlic clove, peeled and finely chopped
1 small red pepper, deseeded and finely sliced
1 small yellow pepper, deseeded and finely sliced
1 tsp granulated sugar
10 ml white wine vinegar
50 ml pork stock
1 tsp tomato purée
1 tbsp light soy sauce
1 tbsp sweet sherry
finely chopped spring onion, to garnish

- *Coat the pork with seasoned flour.*
- *Heat 2 tablespoons of the olive oil in the wok and stir-fry the pork over a medium heat for 4–5 minutes, stirring frequently. Remove the pork with a perforated spoon, set aside and cover.*
- *Heat the remaining tablespoon of olive oil in the wok. Reduce the heat to medium and sauté the spring onions and garlic for about a minute, then add the red and yellow peppers, and stir-fry for 2–3 minutes. Return the pork to the wok, stir in the sugar, white wine vinegar, stock, tomato purée, soy sauce and sherry. Simmer for about 3–4 minutes and serve immediately, garnished with finely chopped spring onion.*

*Carbohydrate content per serving: **21** grams*

Pork with ginger

For 2   250 grams lean pork fillet, sliced thinly on the diagonal
3 tbsp extra-virgin olive oil
1 garlic clove, peeled and finely chopped
3 slices of fresh ginger root, peeled and finely chopped
100 grams mangetout
3 spring onions, chopped into 4–5-cm lengths
1 medium carrot, peeled and chopped into matchsticks
pinch of rock salt
freshly ground black pepper

Marinade

2 tbsp light soy sauce
1 tsp cornflour
2 tbsp dry sherry

* *Mix the soy sauce and sherry in a large bowl and stir in the cornflour to ensure an even consistency. Add the pork and marinate in the fridge for at least 2 hours.*

* *Heat 2 tablespoons of the olive oil in a wok and stir-fry the pork for 2–3 minutes, stirring frequently. Remove the pork with a perforated spoon, set aside and cover.*

* *Heat the remaining tablespoon of olive oil in the wok, add the garlic, ginger, mangetout, spring onions and carrot. Season to taste, stir-fry for 2–3 minutes, then return the pork to the wok. Cook for another 2 minutes and serve immediately.*

*Carbohydrate content per serving: **10** grams*

Pork chops with herbs

For 2   3 tbsp dry white wine
1 garlic clove, peeled and finely chopped
1 tsp chopped fresh sage
1 tsp chopped fresh rosemary
2 large pork chops
2 tbsp extra-virgin olive oil
4 green olives, finely sliced
1 tsp chopped flat-leaf parsley

- *Mix together the white wine, garlic, sage and rosemary, add the pork chops and marinate in the fridge for 3–4 hours.*
- *Heat the olive oil in a large frying pan and cook the pork chops for 2–3 minutes per side on medium heat. Pour the remainder of the marinade over the pork, and cook for another 2–3 minutes, turning once. Garnish with olives and chopped fresh parsley, and serve with cucumber and bean sprout salad (see page 211).*

*Carbohydrate content per serving: **1** gram*

Spicy lamb

For 2   350 grams lean lamb fillet, cubed
         3 tbsp extra-virgin olive oil
         2 green cardamom pods
         1 cinnamon stick
         1 clove
         2 bay leaves
         1 medium onion, peeled and finely sliced
         1 garlic clove, peeled and finely chopped
         2 slices of fresh ginger root, peeled and finely chopped
         1 tbsp chopped fresh coriander
         ½ tsp chilli powder
         ½ tsp ground cumin
         200-gram tin plum tomatoes, chopped into large
             segments
         1 tbsp tomato purée
         150 ml lamb stock

Marinade

         150 ml natural yoghurt
         pinch of rock salt
         freshly ground black pepper
         1 garlic clove, peeled and finely chopped
         1 tbsp freshly squeezed lemon juice

- *Mix together the yoghurt, salt, pepper, garlic and lemon juice. Stir in the lamb and marinate in the fridge for at least 4–6 hours, preferably overnight.*
- *Heat the olive oil in a large frying pan and sauté the cardamom pods, cinnamon stick and clove for about 2 minutes. Add the bay leaf and onion, and sauté until softened. Add the garlic, ginger, coriander, chilli powder and ground cumin, mix well, and cook for*

approximately 2 minutes. Add the lamb to the pan and stir-fry for 4–5 minutes, then add the chopped tomatoes, tomato purée and stock. Bring to the boil, then reduce heat to a gentle simmer. Cover and simmer gently for approximately 1 hour. Remove the bay leaves, cinnamon stick and cardamom pods, and serve with a crispy green salad (see page 209).

*Carbohydrate content per serving: **19** grams*

Lamb skewers with cucumber raita

For 2   300 grams lean minced lamb
1 medium onion, peeled and grated
1 tbsp chopped fresh coriander
1 garlic clove, peeled and grated
1 tbsp chopped fresh flat-leaf parsley
½ tsp ground cumin
½ small green chilli, deseeded and finely chopped
1 egg white, separated
pinch of rock salt
freshly ground black pepper
lime wedges
fresh coriander leaves, to garnish

Cucumber raita

150 ml natural yoghurt
1 tbsp chopped fresh mint leaves
1 small Lebanese cucumber, finely chopped

- Grate the garlic with a ginger- or garlic-grater.
- Mix together the lamb, onion, coriander, garlic, parsley, cumin, chilli, egg white and seasoning (to taste) in a large bowl. Mould the lamb mixture into a sausage shape around kebab sticks, pressing firmly, then cool in the fridge for 2–3 hours. This will help to retain the kebabs' shape whilst grilling.
- Mix the chopped fresh mint and cucumber with the yoghurt, and cool in the fridge for 2–3 hours.
- Remove the kebabs from the fridge and grill on a high heat for 5–7 minutes, turning once. Serve with the mint yoghurt dressing and lime wedges, and garnish with fresh mint leaves.

*Carbohydrate content per serving: **8** grams*

Lamb curry with red pepper

For 2
4 tbsp extra-virgin olive oil
2 medium onions, peeled and chopped
1 garlic clove, peeled and finely chopped
2 small red peppers, deseeded and finely sliced
1 bay leaf
2 green cadamom pods
350 grams lean lamb fillet, cubed
1 tsp garam masala
1 slice fresh ginger root, peeled and finely chopped
1 green chilli, deseeded and finely chopped
1 tbsp freshly squeezed lemon juice
200-gram tin of chopped plum tomatoes (not drained)
200 ml lamb stock
4 tbsp natural yoghurt
1 tbsp fresh coriander, finely chopped
pinch of rock salt
freshly ground black pepper
fresh coriander leaves and slices of red chilli,
    to garnish

- *Heat the extra-virgin olive oil in a large, deep frying pan and sauté the onions, garlic, red peppers, bay leaf and cardamom pods for 1–2 minutes. Add the lamb and sauté for a further 4–5 minutes. Stir in the garam masala, ginger, chilli, lemon juice and tomatoes, and cook for 2–3 minutes. Stir in the stock and simmer gently for 45 minutes. Remove the bay leaf and cardamom pods, then stir in the yoghurt gradually over low heat. Finally, add the fresh coriander, season to taste and simmer over low heat for a further 3–4 minutes. Serve immediately, garnished with fresh coriander leaves and finely sliced red chilli.*

*Carbohydrate content per serving: **16** grams*

Lamb kebabs with soured cream and chive sauce

For 2   300 grams lean lamb fillet, cubed
6 small pickling onions, peeled
6 cherry tomatoes
12 small button mushrooms, wiped
1 yellow pepper, deseeded and chopped into large
    pieces
1 green pepper, deseeded and chopped into large
    pieces
6 skewers
2 tbsp extra-virgin olive oil
freshly ground black pepper
lime wedges

Sauce

100 ml soured cream
50 grams Lebanese cucumber, finely diced
2 tsp chopped fresh chives
1 garlic clove, peeled and finely grated
1 tsp lemon juice

- *Place the soured cream, cucumber, chives, garlic and lemon juice in a medium bowl and mix thoroughly. Chill in the fridge for 2 hours before serving.*
- *Chop the peppers into segments about the size of the lamb cubes, to ensure even cooking times. Thread the lamb cubes, onions, tomatoes, button mushrooms and segments of peppers aesthetically on to 8 skewers. (If wooden skewers are used, remember to soak the skewers in cold water for at least 2 hours before use.)*

- *Brush the lamb and vegetables with the olive oil, season with freshly ground black pepper and grill under a hot grill (or barbecue) for 10–12 minutes, turning frequently. Serve with the chilled soured cream sauce and lime wedges.*

Carbohydrate content per serving: 12 grams

Roast lamb

Roast meats provide delicious hot meals, and equally delicious cold meals the next day. The meat cooks itself with very little preparation, and is really another example of a perfect fast food – except that it is also healthy!

For 4   Leg of lamb (about 1½ kg)
pinch of rock salt
freshly ground black pepper
2 garlic cloves, peeled and sliced
3 tbsp extra-virgin olive oil
2 tbsp chopped fresh rosemary
sprigs of fresh mint to garnish
150 grams French beans
150 grams carrots, peeled and sliced lengthways into matchsticks (Julienne)
150 grams courgettes, Julienne

- *Season the lamb with salt and freshly ground black pepper to taste. Slash the lamb lightly and insert garlic slices into the cuts. Brush the joint with olive oil, sprinkle chopped fresh rosemary over it, place it in a buttered roasting tin and cook in the centre of a pre-heated oven at 220 degrees C (gas mark 7) for 20 minutes. Reduce the temperature to 190 degrees C (gas mark 5) and continue to cook according to the following formula: 20 minutes for each 450 grams, plus an additional 10 minutes. Remove from the oven, allow to cool before carving and garnish with fresh mint.*
- Lightly steam the French beans, carrots and courgettes, and serve with the lamb.

*Carbohydrate content per serving: **9** grams*

Chilli lamb

For 2   250 grams lean lamb fillets, sliced into thin strips
3 tbsp extra-virgin olive oil
1 tsp sesame oil
1 small red chilli, deseeded and finely chopped
3 spring onions, chopped into 4–5-cm lengths
2 slices of fresh ginger root, peeled and grated
1 garlic clove, peeled and finely chopped
1 small red pepper, deseeded and finely sliced
1 small orange pepper, deseeded and finely sliced
50 grams sugar snap peas
2 tbsp light soy sauce
2 green courgettes, chopped on the diagonal
freshly ground black pepper
pinch of rock salt

- *Heat 2 tablespoons of the olive oil in a wok and stir-fry the lamb until tender. Remove from the pan with a perforated spoon, pat dry and set aside to cool.*
- *Heat the remaining olive oil and sesame oil in the wok, add the chilli, spring onions, ginger, garlic, peppers, sugar snap peas and soy sauce, and stir-fry for 1–2 minutes. Return the lamb to the wok, add the courgettes, season to taste, stir-fry for a further 2–3 minutes and serve.*

*Carbohydrate content per serving: **7** grams*

Stir-fried lamb with ginger

For 2   200 grams lean lamb fillet, thinly sliced
         3 tbsp extra-virgin olive oil
         3 spring onions, chopped into 4–5-cm lengths
         1 garlic clove, peeled and finely chopped
         3 slices of fresh ginger root, peeled and finely
           chopped
         1 medium carrot, Julienne
         1 medium yellow pepper, deseeded and finely sliced
         100 grams mangetout
         pinch of rock salt
         freshly ground black pepper

Marinade

         2 tbsp light soy sauce
         1 tbsp dry sherry
         1 tsp granulated sugar
         half a garlic clove, peeled and finely chopped
         1 slice of fresh ginger root, peeled and finely chopped
         2 tsp cornflour

- *In a medium bowl mix together the soy sauce, sherry,
  sugar, garlic and ginger, and gradually stir in the
  cornflour to an even consistency.*
- *Marinate the lamb for 2–3 hours, stirring
  occasionally.*
- *Heat 2 tablespoons of the olive oil in the wok, then
  stir-fry the lamb for 2–3 minutes. Remove with a
  perforated spoon and cover.*
- *Heat the remaining tablespoon of olive oil, add the spring
  onions, garlic, ginger, carrot, pepper and mangetout, and
  stir-fry for 2–3 minutes. Return the lamb to the wok,
  season to taste and stir-fry for a further 2 minutes.*

*Carbohydrate content per serving: **16** grams*

Liver with soured cream

Liver is not a popular dish today, which is incredible when one considers how nutritious and tasty it is. It is packed full of protein, vitamins and minerals; for example, there is 3–4 times more vitamin C in liver than in the equivalent weight of citrus fruits.

For 2
4 thin slices of lamb's liver (approximately 250 grams), sliced into strips
2 tbsp plain flour
1 tbsp paprika
pinch of rock salt
freshly ground black pepper
3 tbsp extra-virgin olive oil
1 large onion, peeled and chopped
1 garlic clove, peeled and finely chopped
200-gram tin of plum tomatoes, chopped
2 tsp tomato purée
150 ml beef stock
2 tsp chopped fresh thyme
2 tsp chopped fresh coriander
2 tsp chopped fresh basil
100 ml soured cream
sprigs of fresh thyme, to garnish

- *Mix the flour with the paprika and season with salt and freshly ground black pepper. Coat the liver in the seasoned flour. Heat the extra-virgin olive oil in a frying pan and brown the liver. Add the onion and garlic and sauté for about 1 minute. Add the tomatoes, tomato purée, stock and herbs, stirring constantly. Season to taste and simmer for about 30 minutes. Stir in the soured cream and serve immediately, garnished with sprigs of fresh basil.*

*Carbohydrate content per serving: **21** grams*

Braised liver with mushrooms

For 2   2 tbsp plain flour
pinch of rock salt
freshly ground black pepper
4 thin slices of lamb's liver (approximately 250 grams)
4 tbsp extra-virgin olive oil
1 garlic clove, peeled and finely chopped
1 large onion, peeled and chopped
1 tbsp sweet sherry
150 grams button mushrooms, wiped and halved
1 bay leaf
sprigs of fresh thyme, to garnish

- *Season the flour with the salt and black pepper and coat the liver with it.*
- *Heat 3 tablespoons of the olive oil in a frying pan, then cook the liver for about 6 minutes, turning once. Remove with a perforated spoon to a shallow dish, cover and place in a warm oven. Heat the remaining tablespoon of olive oil in the pan and sauté the onion and garlic for about a minute. Add the sherry, mushrooms and bay leaf, and sauté for a further 2 minutes.*
- *Return the liver to the pan and cook on medium heat for 2 minutes, turning once. Remove the bay leaf and serve, garnished with fresh thyme.*

*Carbohydrate content per serving: **16** grams*

Liver casserole

For 2
2 tbsp plain flour
pinch of rock salt
freshly ground black pepper
3–4 slices of lamb's liver (about 250–300 grams)
3 tbsp extra-virgin olive oil
1 medium onion, peeled and finely sliced
1 garlic clove, peeled and finely chopped
1 green pepper, deseeded and chopped into large
    segments
1 large carrot, peeled and sliced on the diagonal
3 tbsp dry white wine
200 ml lamb stock
1 tsp chopped fresh thyme
1 tsp chopped fresh flat-leaf parsley

- *Season the flour with the salt and black pepper and
  coat the liver with it.*
- *Heat 2 tablespoons of olive oil in a large pan and
  brown the liver. Remove the liver with a perforated
  spoon, place in a casserole dish and cover.*
- *Add the remaining tablespoon of olive oil to the pan
  and sauté the onion and garlic for approximately 1
  minute. Add the green pepper and carrot, and sauté for
  a further 2 minutes, stirring frequently. Stir in the wine
  and stock, chopped fresh thyme and parsley, and
  season to taste. Transfer to the casserole dish, cover
  and cook in a pre-heated oven at 140 degrees C (gas
  mark 1), for about 2–2½ hours, depending on the oven.*

*Carbohydrate content per serving: **20** grams*

Lamb's liver with herbs

For 2   3 tbsp extra-virgin olive oil
1 medium red onion, peeled and diced
1 garlic clove, peeled and finely chopped
4 thin slices of lamb's liver (approximately 250 grams)
2 tbsp plain flour
pinch of rock salt
freshly ground black pepper
200-gram tin of plum tomatoes
1 tbsp chopped fresh oregano
1 tbsp chopped fresh basil
1 tbsp chopped fresh chives
100 grams sugar snap peas
100 grams yellow squash

- *Heat 2 tablespoons of the extra-virgin olive oil in a large frying pan and sauté the onion and garlic for 1–2 minutes.*
- *Coat the liver with seasoned flour, heat the remaining olive oil and cook the liver for 5–6 minutes on medium heat, turning once. Add the tomatoes, oregano and basil, season to taste, and simmer for 5–7 minutes.*
- *Serve with lightly steamed sugar snap peas and yellow squash, garnished with chopped fresh chives.*

*Carbohydrate content per serving: **22** grams*

Chapter 12 Poultry

Tandoori-style chicken

For 2
 2 skinless chicken breasts (about 150 grams each),
   or 6 chicken drumsticks, skin removed
 100 ml natural yoghurt
 1 garlic clove, peeled and grated
 1 slice of fresh ginger root, peeled and grated
 1 tsp garam masala
 1 tsp ground paprika
 ½ tsp ground turmeric
 ½ tsp ground coriander
 ¼ tsp ground cumin
 2 tbsp freshly squeezed lemon juice
 pinch of rock salt
 freshly ground black pepper
 lemon wedges

- *Cut two slits in each of the chicken pieces (breast or drumsticks). Mix the yoghurt with the garlic, ginger, spices, lemon juice and seasoning, and coat the chicken with the sauce. Marinate in the fridge for at least 4 hours (preferably overnight).*
- *Lay the chicken in a single layer on an oven tray, cover with pierced aluminium foil and cook in the centre of a pre-heated oven for 30–35 minutes at 180 degrees C (gas mark 4), turning once.*
- *Serve with a crispy green salad (see page 209) and lemon wedges.*

*Carbohydrate content per serving: **11** grams*

Chicken tikka

A delicious dish, not too spicy, which combines the natural proteins, vitamins and minerals of the chicken with the vitamins and antioxidants of the herbs.

For 2   300 grams skinless chicken breast, cubed

Marinade

½ tsp chilli powder
1 garlic clove, peeled and finely chopped
2 slices fresh ginger root, peeled and finely chopped
½ tsp ground turmeric
½ tsp ground cumin
1 shallot, peeled and grated
pinch of rock salt
freshly ground black pepper
2 tsp fresh lemon juice
100 ml natural yoghurt
2 tsp fresh coriander, finely chopped

- *Mix together the chilli powder, garlic, ginger, turmeric, cumin, shallot, salt, pepper, lemon juice, natural yoghurt and coriander in a medium bowl, and stir in the chicken. Cover and leave to marinate in the fridge for at least 3–4 hours – or preferably overnight.*
- *Grill the marinated chicken under medium heat for about 20 minutes, turning regularly.*
- *Serve with a crispy green salad (see page 209) and lime wedges.*

*Carbohydrate content per serving: **11** grams*

Lemon chicken with cashew nuts

For 2   3 tbsp extra-virgin olive oil
250 grams skinless chicken breast, thinly sliced
50 grams raw cashew nuts
lemon wedges
75 grams mangetout
75 grams broccoli florets
lemon zest, to garnish

Sauce

1 tsp cornflour
2 tbsp water
juice of a freshly squeezed lemon
1 tbsp light soy sauce
2 tbsp sweet sherry

- *Prepare the cornflour mixture by adding the cornflour to 2 tablespoons of water, stirring to ensure an even consistency.*
- *Heat the olive oil in the wok, then stir-fry the chicken breast strips on medium heat for about 3–4 minutes, stirring frequently. Remove the chicken to a casserole dish, mix with the cashew nuts, cover and place in a warm oven. Drain the wok and wipe clean.*
- *Mix together the lemon juice, soy sauce and sherry in a bowl, and stir in the cornflour paste, mixing to an even consistency. Transfer to the wok and heat to a gentle simmer, stirring constantly for about 1–2 minutes, until the sauce thickens.*
- *Return the chicken and cashew nuts to the wok and simmer for 2–3 minutes.*
- *Lightly steam the mangetout and broccoli florets. Garnish the chicken with lemon zest and serve with the vegetables.*

Carbohydrate content per serving: **15** *grams*

Chicken with prosciutto

The cheese in this recipe can be varied according to taste – it is equally delicious with Edam, Emmental, Gruyère or Jarlsberg. I consider strong cheeses (such as mature Cheddar and Stilton) to be too overpowering for this combination. If you are partial to cheeses with strong flavour (which I think are wonderful in other circumstances), then simply reduce the quantity.

For 2
- 2 skinless chicken breast fillets (about 150 grams each)
- 2 tbsp plain flour, seasoned
- 2 tbsp extra-virgin olive oil
- 1 tbsp fresh basil, finely chopped
- 4 large slices of prosciutto (sliced)
- 30 grams freshly grated Parmesan cheese
- freshly ground black pepper
- 1 tsp chopped fresh chives, to garnish
- 1 tsp chopped fresh coriander, to garnish

- *Using a sharp knife, slice each chicken breast lengthways into two thin, flat halves. Season the flour with salt and black pepper and lightly coat the chicken breasts with it.*
- *Heat the olive oil in a frying pan, add the chicken fillets and chopped basil, and cook over a moderate heat for 8–10 minutes, turning twice, until evenly cooked on both sides. Remove the chicken to a grill-pan, place a slice of prosciutto on each fillet, and sprinkle grated Parmesan cheese on the prosciutto. Season with freshly ground black pepper and place under a pre-heated grill until the cheese has just melted.*
- *Serve with tomato and avocado salad (see page 204), garnished with fresh chives and coriander.*

*Carbohydrate content per serving: **20** grams (including salad)*

Chicken korma

For 2

300 grams skinless chicken breasts, cubed
3 tbsp extra-virgin olive oil
2 green cardamom pods
1 medium onion, peeled and finely chopped
1 garlic clove, peeled and finely chopped
1 slice of fresh ginger root, peeled and finely chopped
1 tsp ground cumin
½ tsp garam masala
½ tsp chilli powder
pinch of rock salt
freshly ground black pepper
125 ml natural yoghurt
pinch of paprika and some fresh coriander leaves, to garnish

- *Heat 2 tablespoons of the olive oil in a large frying pan and sauté the chicken for 5–6 minutes, stirring frequently. Remove the chicken with a perforated spoon, place it in a casserole dish and cover.*
- *Heat the remaining tablespoon of olive oil in the pan, add the cardamom pods, onion and garlic, and sauté for 2–3 minutes. Remove from the heat and stir in the ginger, cumin, garam masala, chilli powder and seasoning. Cook over a low heat for 2–3 minutes, stirring constantly. Stir in the yoghurt gradually, simmer over low heat for 2–3 minutes, then return the chicken to the pan. Heat through gently for about 3–4 minutes, then serve, garnished with a pinch of paprika and some fresh coriander leaves.*

*Carbohydrate content per serving: **7** grams*

Chicken with tomato and basil sauce

For 2
2 skinless chicken breasts (about 150 grams each)
25 grams butter, cubed
3 tbsp extra-virgin olive oil
1 medium onion, peeled and chopped
1 garlic clove, peeled and finely chopped
400-gram tin of plum tomatoes
1 tbsp tomato purée
50 ml dry white wine
75 ml chicken stock
75 grams button mushrooms, wiped and halved
1 tbsp chopped fresh basil
pinch of rock salt
freshly ground black pepper
100 grams broccoli florets
100 grams carrots, julienned
fresh basil leaves, to garnish

- *Place the chicken breasts in the base of a shallow roasting tray, arrange the cubes of butter on the chicken, then cover with pierced aluminium foil and cook in centre of a pre-heated oven at 180 degrees C (gas mark 4) for 35–40 minutes. Remove the fillets with a perforated spoon and allow to cool, then chop into large cubes.*
- *Heat the olive oil in a large frying pan and sauté the onion and garlic for 1–2 minutes. Add the tomatoes, tomato purée, red wine, stock and mushrooms, then simmer for 6–8 minutes. Stir in the chopped basil and chicken, season to taste and simmer for a further 15 minutes.*
- *Lightly steam the broccoli and carrots. Garnish the chicken with fresh basil leaves and serve.*

*Carbohydrate content per serving: **17** grams*

Chicken burritos

If time is short, you can omit the guacamole from this recipe. Remember, if you are in the active weight-loss phase of the diet, you must have no more than one slice of bread or one tortilla per day.

For 2
200 grams skinless chicken breast
25 grams butter, cubed
2 medium flour tortillas
2 tbsp tomato salsa (see page 225)
100 ml shredded sweet romaine lettuce
100 grams guacamole (see page 203)
50 grams freshly grated Emmental (or mild Cheddar, such as Orkney or Bute)
freshly ground black pepper

- *Place the skinless chicken breasts in a shallow, oven-safe dish, top with butter cubes, cover with pierced aluminium foil and cook in the centre of a pre-heated oven at 180 degrees C (gas mark 4) for 35–40 minutes. Remove with a perforated spoon and set aside to cool, then slice thinly. If preferred, the chicken breasts can be grilled or fried, according to taste, without affecting the diet in any way.*
- *Allow the chicken slices to cool and then mix them with the salsa.*
- *Wrap the tortillas in aluminium foil and place in a hot oven for 1 minute. Remove from the oven, spoon the chicken salsa mixture into the centre of each tortilla, top with shredded lettuce, guacamole and freshly grated cheese of your choice (but Emmental is ideal for this recipe). Season with freshly ground black pepper, and fold the tortilla over to close.*

Carbohydrate content per serving: **33–38** grams (only **8–13** grams without the tortilla)

Tarragon chicken with tomato and avocado

For 2   250–300 grams skinless chicken breast
         75 ml mayonnaise (to make your own see page 116,
              or a ready-made brand)
         1 tbsp chopped fresh tarragon
         pinch of rock salt
         freshly ground black pepper
         tomato and avocado salad (see page 204)
         sprigs of fresh tarragon, to garnish

- *Bake the chicken as described on page 178, allow to cool, then slice thinly.*
- *Stir the chopped tarragon into the mayonnaise and season to taste. Arrange the chicken slices on the plate and top with the tarragon mayonnaise. Serve with the tomato and avocado salad, garnished with sprigs of fresh tarragon.*

Carbohydrate content per serving: 8 grams (including salad)

Roast duck with juniper berries and orange liqueur sauce

For 4   2 tbsp fresh juniper berries, crushed
pinch of rock salt
freshly ground black pepper
50 grams butter
1 oven-ready duck (2.5–3 kg)
150 grams carrots, julienne
150 grams yellow squash
150 grams mangetout

Sauce

50 grams unsalted butter
2 tsp cornflour
200 ml chicken stock
1 tbsp freshly squeezed lemon juice
3 tbsp freshly squeezed orange juice
1 tbsp sweet sherry
50 ml Cointreau

- *Mix the crushed juniper berries, salt and freshly ground black pepper in a bowl, and transfer to a plate. Rub the butter over the duck, then roll the duck in the juniper berry mixture. Prick the duck skin liberally with a skewer. Place the duck on a rack in a roasting tin to allow the excess fat to drain as the duck is cooking, and cook at 220 degrees C (gas mark 7) for 20 minutes, then reduce the heat to 180 degrees C (gas mark 4) and cook for 2½–3 hours (depending on the size of the duck), basting once. Remove from the oven and allow to cool.*
- *Lightly steam the carrots, squash and mangetout until tender but still firm.*
- *While the duck is cooking, prepare the sauce. Melt*

the butter in a small saucepan, remove from the heat and gradually stir in the cornflour to form a smooth paste. Stir in the stock to an even consistency, then return to the heat and simmer gently. Stir in the lemon juice, orange juice and sherry over a low simmer. Add the Cointreau when the sauce thickens. Remove from the heat, continuing to stir.

- Carve the duck and serve with the carrots, yellow squash and mangetout, and – of course – the orange liqueur sauce.

Carbohydrate content per serving: 21 grams

Chapter 13 Eggs

As I have already mentioned, eggs provide many of the proteins, vitamins and minerals essential for good health. They are also an excellent source of cysteine, the amino acid essential for the production of a major antioxidant enzyme, glutathione.

Eggs can form the basis of a meal at any time of day; the following recipes can be eaten for breakfast, brunch, lunch or supper, the only difference being that some take a little longer than others, or may be more savoury. Eggs certainly don't have to be included in your diet every day – and don't have to included at all if you don't like eggs. They should only be used in one meal per day at the most – so if you've had eggs for breakfast, don't have eggs for supper.

Piperade

For 2   50 grams butter
1 small red pepper, deseeded and diced
1 small yellow pepper, deseeded and diced
1 small onion, peeled and finely chopped
1 garlic clove, peeled and finely chopped
2 large fresh plum tomatoes, skinned, seeded and diced
pinch of rock salt
freshly ground black pepper
4 large free-range eggs
2 tbsp full-cream milk
1 tsp fresh coriander, finely chopped
black olives, chopped, to garnish (optional)

- *Melt the butter and sauté the peppers, onion and garlic for about 3–4 minutes. Add the tomatoes, season to taste and cook for another 2 minutes.*
- *Whisk the eggs with the milk and pour over the vegetables. Add the chopped coriander, stirring gently until the mixture just sets but is still creamy, and serve immediately, garnished with chopped black olives.*

Carbohydrate content per serving: **7** *grams*

Smoked salmon with creamy eggs
This is a very rich dish. Three large eggs therefore provide a
satisfying meal for two.

For 2   3 large free-range eggs
2 tbsp single cream
freshly ground black pepper
25 grams unsalted butter
50 grams smoked salmon, finely sliced
2 tsp chopped fresh dill
pinch of paprika

- *Beat together the eggs and 1 tablespoon of the
  cream, and season with freshly ground black pepper
  (salt is not really necessary for this dish as smoked
  salmon is naturally salty). Melt the butter in a small
  saucepan and scramble the eggs lightly. When the
  eggs have almost set but are still creamy, mix in the
  smoked salmon and the remaining cream, gently heat
  through and serve on warm plates, garnished with
  chopped fresh dill and a pinch of paprika.*

Carbohydrate content per serving: negligible

Prosciutto and courgette frittata

For 2   50 grams butter

1 small onion, peeled and diced

1 garlic clove, peeled and finely chopped

1 small red pepper, deseeded and thinly sliced

1 medium courgette, thinly sliced

4 large free-range eggs

50 ml full-cream milk

pinch of rock salt

freshly ground black pepper

2 tsp Worcestershire sauce

100 grams freshly grated cheese. Italian cheeses
such as Parmesan or Fontina are ideal, but this
dish can readily adapt to individual taste. Gruyère,
Emmental, Edam or even stronger cheeses such as
Wensleydale are equally effective

pinch of rock salt

freshly ground black pepper

2 thin slices of prosciutto, finely shredded

- *Melt the butter in a medium frying pan and sauté the onion, garlic and red pepper for about 2 minutes. Add the courgette, and sauté for a further 2–3 minutes, until soft but firm.*
- *Beat the eggs and milk together with the salt, freshly ground pepper and Worcestershire sauce in a bowl, then mix in 75 grams of grated cheese. Pour the mixture over the vegetables, stirring gently to cover the base of the pan with the egg mixture.*
- *Cook over a very low heat until the mixture just sets, which usually takes about 10 minutes. Sprinkle the shredded ham over the frittata, then top with grated cheese to ensure that all of the ham is covered. Place*

> *under a hot grill for about 30–40 seconds, or until the cheese has just melted.*
> • *Remove from the heat, allow the frittata to cool, then remove from the pan with a palette knife and halve. Serve with crispy green salad (see page 209) or rocket and avocado salad (see page 213).*

*Carbohydrate content per serving: **13** grams with green salad, **8** grams with rocket salad*

Baked eggs with lemon cream sauce and chives

For 2 2 large free-range eggs
75 ml single cream
1 tbsp freshly squeezed lemon juice
freshly ground black pepper
1 tbsp chopped fresh chives and ground paprika, to
    garnish

> • *Butter 2 ramekins, gently break an egg into each one and bake in a pre-heated oven at 180 degrees C (gas mark 4) for 7–8 minutes (depending on the size of the eggs).*
> • *While the eggs are baking, gently heat the cream in a small saucepan and gradually stir in the lemon juice. Season with freshly ground black pepper.*
> • *Remove the eggs from the oven, pour the lemon sauce over the eggs, and garnish with chopped chives and ground paprika. Serve with tomato and avocado salad (see page 204).*

*Carbohydrate content per serving: **9** grams*

Chicken and pepper frittata

Frittata is so delicious cold the next day that I always make extra for additional snacks or meals.

For 4   2 chicken breasts, about 150 grams each
          25 grams butter, cubed
          2 tbsp extra-virgin olive oil
          1 red onion, peeled and diced
          1 garlic clove, peeled and finely chopped
          1 small green pepper, deseeded and finely sliced
          1 small yellow pepper, deseeded and finely sliced
          6 large free-range eggs, beaten
          pinch of rock salt
          freshly ground black pepper
          50 grams freshly grated Gruyère

- *Place the chicken breast fillets in a shallow oven-safe dish, top with cubes of butter, cover with pierced aluminium foil and cook in the centre of a pre-heated oven at 180 degrees C (gas mark 4) for 35–40 minutes. Remove the chicken with a perforated spoon, allow to cool, then slice into thin strips.*
- *Heat the olive oil in a medium frying pan and sauté the onion and garlic for about 1 minute. Add the peppers and sauté for a further 3–4 minutes, then return the chicken to the pan, add the eggs and season to taste. Stir in the Gruyère cheese and cook over a low heat until just set. Place under the grill for 30–40 seconds to lightly brown, and serve.*

*Carbohydrate content per serving: **6** grams*

Scrambled eggs and asparagus

For 2 3 large free-range eggs
2 tbsp full-cream milk
25 grams butter
pinch of rock salt
freshly ground black pepper
50 grams freshly grated Jarlsberg
100 grams fresh asparagus
1 tbsp chopped fresh chives, to garnish

- *Scramble the eggs (see pages 68–9) until they are just beginning to set but still creamy. Season to taste, transfer to a small shallow grill-safe dish and top with freshly grated Jarlsberg cheese. Place under a hot grill until the cheese has just melted.*
- *In the meantime, lightly steam the asparagus until just tender.*
- *Arrange the asparagus on warm plates, top with cheesy scrambled eggs, and garnish with chopped fresh chives.*

*Carbohydrate content per serving: **2** grams*

Poached egg with Swiss cheese

For 2   2 large free-range eggs
50 grams freshly grated Emmental
freshly ground black pepper
2 slices buttered wholemeal toast

- *Poach the eggs, then remove from the boiling water with a perforated spoon and place on a slice of hot, buttered wholemeal toast. Sprinkle with the Emmental and place under a hot grill until the cheese melts. Add freshly ground black pepper to taste.*

Carbohydrate content per serving: **17** *grams (or 'nil', without the toast)*

....

Creamed spinach eggs with smoked mackerel

For 2   4 large fresh organic eggs
25 grams butter
50 grams chopped spinach leaves, stalks removed
2 tbsp crème fraîche
150 grams smoked mackerel
freshly ground black pepper

- *Beat the eggs in a medium bowl.*
- *Melt the butter in a medium saucepan over a low heat, add the eggs and allow them to set.*
- *Stir in the spinach, crème fraîche and smoked mackerel.*
- *Serve immediately, seasoned with freshly ground black pepper.*

Carbohydrate content per serving: **3** *grams*

Egg rolls with Jarlsberg and sun-dried tomatoes

For 2
4 large fresh organic eggs
2 tbsp extra-virgin olive oil
60 grams Jarlsberg cheese, grated
2 sun-dried tomatoes, finely chopped
freshly ground black pepper
1 tbsp chopped fresh chives

- *Beat the eggs in a mixing bowl.*
- *Heat the extra-virgin olive oil in a large frying pan and add about a quarter of the egg mixture.*
- *Allow the egg to set (approximately 2 minutes).*
- *Remove from the heat, and place about a quarter of the cheese and tomatoes on the egg roll.*
- *Season to taste and roll into a cylindrical shape.*
- *Repeat the process to make 3 more egg rolls.*
- *Garnish with chopped fresh chives and serve immediately.*

*Carbohydrate content per serving: **3** grams*

Emmental soufflé

For 2   50 grams unsalted butter
1 ½ tbsp plain flour
pinch of dry mustard powder
150 ml full-cream milk
50 grams Emmental cheese, grated
4 large organic free-range eggs, separated
2 tsp grated Parmesan cheese
freshly ground black pepper

- *Heat the butter in a medium saucepan and stir in the flour and mustard to form a roux.*
- *Remove from the heat and gradually stir in the milk.*
- *Return to the heat, stirring constantly, until the mixture just begins to thicken.*
- *Remove from the heat and stir in the Emmental and egg yolks and season to taste with freshly ground black pepper.*
- *Beat the egg whites in a medium mixing bowl, then gradually fold them into the mixture.*
- *Pour the mixture into a soufflé dish and sprinkle with the Parmesan cheese.*
- *Cook in the centre of a preheated oven at 180 degrees C (gas mark 4) for about 20–25 minutes.*

*Carbohydrate content per serving: **15** grams*

Chapter 14 Vegetable dishes

Leeks and lemon hollandaise sauce

For 2 8 baby leeks
pinch of rock salt
freshly ground black pepper
4 tbsp lemon hollandaise sauce (see page 110)

- *Season the leeks and lightly steam until tender but still firm. Remove with a perforated spoon, place on warm plates and pour the sauce over.*

Carbohydrate content per serving: 6 grams

Char-grilled vegetables with oregano

For 2
1 medium red pepper, deseeded and chopped into large pieces

1 medium yellow pepper, deseeded and chopped into large pieces

6 baby onions, peeled and halved

1 courgette, sliced lengthways

6 cherry tomatoes

2 tbsp extra-virgin olive oil

pinch of rock salt

freshly ground black pepper

fresh oregano leaves to garnish

Dressing

4 tbsp extra-virgin olive oil

1 tbsp balsamic vinegar

1 tsp freshly squeezed lemon juice

2 tsp chopped fresh oregano

freshly ground black pepper

- *Place the dressing ingredients in a screw-top jar and shake until thoroughly mixed.*
- *Arrange the vegetables in a single layer, skin uppermost, on a shallow grill-safe buttered baking tray, brush with extra-virgin olive oil and grill under medium heat for 5–6 minutes, turning frequently. Remove from the grill, peel the skin from the peppers and onion, and transfer to warm plates. Drizzle the dressing over the vegetables, season to taste and serve garnished with fresh oregano leaves.*

Carbohydrate content per serving: **8** *grams*

Ratatouille

For 2

1 medium aubergine, cubed
pinch of rock salt
3 tbsp extra-virgin olive oil
2 courgettes, chopped
1 medium red pepper, deseeded and chopped
1 medium yellow pepper, deseeded and chopped
1 large onion, peeled and sliced
1 garlic clove, peeled and finely chopped
3 large plum tomatoes, peeled and chopped
75 ml tomato juice
1 tbsp tomato purée
pinch of granulated sugar
1 bay leaf
1 tbsp chopped fresh basil
1 tsp chopped fresh oregano
freshly ground black pepper
fresh basil leaves, to garnish

- *Place the chopped aubergine into a colander, sprinkle with salt, allow to stand for 20–30 minutes, then rinse with cold water and pat dry.*
- *Heat 2 tablespoons of the extra-virgin olive oil in a large frying pan (or preferably a wok) until hot, add the aubergine, courgettes and peppers, and sauté for 2 minutes. Remove with a perforated spoon and cover.*
- *Heat the remaining tablespoon of olive oil in the pan and sauté the onion and garlic. Add the tomatoes, tomato juice, tomato purée, sugar and bay leaf; return the aubergine, courgettes and peppers to the pan, and stir in the basil and oregano. Season to taste and gently simmer for about 6–7 minutes. Remove the bay leaf and serve, garnished with fresh basil leaves.*

Carbohydrate content per serving: **16 grams**

Baked fennel with basil and Gruyère

For 2   3 fennel bulbs, peeled
        25 grams butter, cubed
        1 tbsp chopped fresh basil
        pinch of rock salt
        freshly ground black pepper
        50 grams freshly grated Gruyère
        fresh basil leaves, to garnish

- *Place the fennel (in a single layer) in the base of a large saucepan. Add only sufficient water to almost cover, then bring to the boil and simmer until the fennel just softens.*
- *Remove with a perforated spoon and halve the fennel bulbs lengthways. Place in the base of a shallow oven-safe dish in a single layer, and sprinkle with chopped basil and cubes of butter. Season to taste, and top with a layer of Gruyère. Bake in the centre of a pre-heated oven at 180 degrees C (gas mark 4) for 10 minutes and serve, garnished with fresh basil leaves.*

Carbohydrate content per serving: 4 grams

Stir-fried vegetables

For 2   3 tbsp extra-virgin olive oil
1 garlic clove, peeled and finely chopped
2 slices of fresh ginger root, peeled and finely
    chopped
75 grams broccoli florets
3 spring onions, chopped into 4–5-cm lengths
1 medium red pepper, deseeded and finely sliced
1 medium yellow pepper, deseeded and finely sliced
100 grams mangetout
50 grams button mushrooms, wiped and halved
2 tbsp light soy sauce
2 tbsp sweet sherry
pinch of rock salt
freshly ground black pepper

- *Heat the olive oil in a wok, sauté the garlic and ginger for about 30 seconds, then add the broccoli, spring onions, peppers, mangetout, mushrooms, soy sauce and sherry. Season to taste and stir-fry over medium heat for 3–4 minutes, then serve immediately.*

Carbohydrate content per serving: **12** *grams*

Cauliflower and asparagus frittata

For 2 half a small cauliflower, cut into florets
100 grams asparagus, cut into 2-cm segments
  diagonally
2 tbsp extra-virgin olive oil
2 shallots, peeled and diced
1 garlic clove, peeled and finely chopped
4 large free-range eggs, beaten
freshly ground black pepper
25 grams Parmesan cheese, freshly grated

- *Lightly steam the cauliflower and asparagus for
  10 minutes (or cook in the microwave on high for
  3 minutes).*
- *Set aside to cool.*
- *Heat the olive oil in a medium frying pan and sauté
  the shallots and garlic for 1 minute.*
- *Add the eggs, mix in the cauliflower and asparagus
  and season to taste.*
- *Cook over a low heat until just set.*
- *Sprinkle over the Parmesan cheese and place under
  a medium grill for 30–40 seconds to lightly brown.*
- *Serve immediately.*

*Carbohydrate content per serving: **7** grams*

Tofu kebabs with satay sauce

For 2   100 grams tofu, chopped into 2-cm cubes

75 grams button mushrooms, washed

1 small red pepper, deseeded and chopped
   into 2-cm cubes

1 small green pepper, deseeded and chopped
   into 2-cm cubes

2 courgettes, chopped

freshly ground black pepper

1 tbsp chopped fresh coriander leaves

Satay sauce (page 219)

Marinade

2 tbsp soy sauce

2 tbsp dry sherry

2 slices fresh ginger, peeled and grated

1 small garlic clove, peeled and grated

- Mix together the marinade ingredients and marinate the cubed tofu for 4 hours in the fridge.

At the same time

- *Soak some satay skewers in cold water.*
- *Thread the tofu, mushrooms, peppers and courgettes alternately onto the satay sticks, drizzle over the marinade and cook under a grill (no closer than 8–10 cm) for 8 minutes, turning occasionally.*
- *Season to taste, top with fresh coriander leaves and serve with satay sauce.*

*Carbohydrate content per serving: **12** grams*

Mint peas

For 2   300 grams fresh peas
50 grams butter
3 spring onions, trimmed and chopped diagonally
50 grams baby spinach leaves
chopped fresh mint leaves, to taste
pinch of rock salt
freshly ground black pepper

- *Shell the peas.*
- *Melt the butter in a medium-sized saucepan over a gentle heat.*
- *Gently sauté the spring onions, spinach and peas for several minutes.*
- *Stir in the fresh mint, cook for a further minute and serve immediately, seasoned with black pepper to taste.*

*Carbohydrate content per serving: **14** grams*

Sweet chilli broccoli

For 2
150 grams broccoli florets
1 tbsp sweet chilli sauce
freshly ground black pepper

- *Microwave the broccoli florets for 2 minutes on high (or steam for 4–5 minutes).*
- *Mix with the sweet chilli sauce.*
- *Serve immediately, seasoned with freshly ground black pepper.*

Carbohydrate content per serving: **3** *grams*

Stir-fried kale with soy sauce

For 2
2 tbsp extra-virgin olive oil
100 grams fresh kale, chopped
2 tsp soy sauce
freshly ground black pepper

- Heat the extra-virgin olive oil in a wok.
- Add the kale and stir-fry for 2–3 minutes.
- Stir in the soy sauce.
- Serve immediately, seasoned with freshly ground black pepper.

Carbohydrate content per serving: **4** *grams*

Leeks and mozzarella

For 2   30 grams unsalted butter
2 large leeks, sliced into rounds
1 medium red onion, peeled and chopped finely
50 grams mozzarella, sliced
1 tbsp chopped fresh oregano
4 slices pancetta, chopped
freshly ground black pepper

- *Melt the butter in a large frying pan and gently fry the leeks, onion and pancetta until soft.*
- *Top with mozzarella and oregano and place under a medium grill (no closer than 8–10 cm) until the mozzarella melts.*
- *Season to taste with freshly ground black pepper and serve immediately.*

Carbohydrate content per serving: **4 grams**

Chapter 15 Salads

Guacamole

For 2

1 large ripe Hass avocado, halved, stoned, peeled and finely diced
½ garlic clove, peeled and finely grated
½ a small onion, peeled and finely chopped
½ ripe plum tomato, peeled, seeded and finely chopped
½ a fresh green chilli, deseeded and finely chopped
2 tsp freshly squeezed lime juice
1 tbsp crème fraîche
freshly ground black pepper

- *Blend together the avocado, garlic, onion, tomato, chilli, lime juice and crème fraîche. Season to taste and chill before serving.*

*Carbohydrate content per serving: **5** grams*

Tomato and avocado salad

For 2   1 medium, ripe Hass avocado, halved, stoned, peeled
and diced
2 tsp freshly squeezed lemon juice
4 large vine-ripened tomatoes, chopped
1 small yellow pepper, deseeded and sliced
1 medium red onion, peeled and sliced into thin rings
freshly ground black pepper

Vinaigrette

4 tbsp extra-virgin olive oil
1 tbsp balsamic vinegar
pinch of rock salt
freshly ground black pepper

- *Add the extra-virgin olive oil, balsamic vinegar, salt
and freshly ground black pepper to a screw-top jar
and mix thoroughly.*
- *Mix the avocado with the lemon juice, then add the
tomatoes and onion. Season to taste and drizzle the
balsamic vinaigrette over the salad.*

*Carbohydrate content per serving: **8** grams*

Feta salad

For 2   ½ a cos lettuce, washed and leaves separated
3 plum tomatoes, chopped
3 spring onions, chopped into 4–5-cm lengths
1 small Lebanese cucumber, sliced lengthways
1 small yellow pepper, deseeded and sliced
50 grams feta cheese, cubed
25 grams black olives

Vinaigrette

4 tbsp extra-virgin olive oil
1 tbsp white wine vinegar
pinch of rock salt
freshly ground black pepper

- *Mix the salad ingredients in a large bowl.*
- *Place the olive oil, white wine vinegar, salt and freshly ground black pepper in a screw-top jar and mix thoroughly. Toss the salad and drizzle the dressing over.*

*Carbohydrate content per serving: **16** grams*

Tomato and coriander salsa

For 2   4 large plum tomatoes, chopped
3 spring onions, finely chopped
½ a small green chilli, deseeded and finely chopped
1 tbsp chopped fresh coriander
pinch of rock salt
freshly ground black pepper
vinaigrette (see page 225)
sprigs of fresh coriander, to garnish

• *Mix together the tomatoes, onion, chilli and chopped coriander, and season to taste. Drizzle the vinaigrette over the salsa and garnish with fresh coriander.*

Carbohydrate content per serving: **7** *grams*

Bocconcini and avocado salad

For 2   2 cherry tomatoes
1 small ripe Hass avocado, halved, stoned, peeled and finely sliced
100 grams Bocconcini cheese, finely sliced
freshly ground black pepper
1 tbsp chopped fresh basil leaves
balsamic vinaigrette (see page 220)

• *Place a cherry tomato in the centre of each plate and arrange the slices of avocado around the tomato like the spokes of a wheel. Arrange the Bocconcini slices on the avocado, season with freshly ground black pepper, garnish with chopped basil leaves and drizzle the balsamic vinaigrette over the salad.*

Carbohydrate content per serving: **2** *grams*

Tomato and Parmesan salad

For 2 6 large plum tomatoes, chopped into big chunks
8 black olives
freshly ground black pepper
1 tbsp chopped fresh chives
balsamic vinaigrette (see page 220)
75 grams freshly grated Parmesan
sprigs of fresh basil, to garnish

- *Mix together the chopped tomatoes and olives, and place on a shallow dish. Season with freshly ground black pepper and sprinkle the chopped fresh chives over. Drizzle over the dressing, sprinkle with freshly grated Parmesan, and garnish with sprigs of fresh basil.*

*Carbohydrate content per serving: **9** grams*

Char-grilled pepper salad with herb mayonnaise

For 2
1 medium red pepper, deseeded and quartered
1 medium green pepper, deseeded and quartered
1 medium yellow pepper, deseeded and quartered
1 red onion, peeled and quartered
1 fennel bulb, peeled and quartered
2 tbsp extra-virgin olive oil
handful of red oak leaf lettuce leaves
fresh coriander leaves, to garnish

Herb mayonnaise
1 tbsp chopped fresh thyme
1 tbsp chopped fresh parsley
1 tsp chopped fresh coriander
100 ml mayonnaise (see page 116)

- *Mix the chopped fresh parsley and thyme into the mayonnaise.*
- *Place the peppers (skin uppermost), onion and fennel quarters in a single layer on a grill tray. Brush with olive oil and cook under a pre-heated grill for about 5 minutes, or until the skin of the peppers blisters. Peel the peppers and remove the outer skin of the onion and fennel, then slice them into thin strips and allow to cool. Arrange the vegetables on a bed of red oak leaf lettuce leaves in a shallow dish, top with the herb mayonnaise and garnish with fresh coriander leaves.*

*Carbohydrate content per serving: **11** grams*

Crispy green salad

For 2   100 grams mixed crispy lettuce leaves (cos, curly
endive, coral, green oak leaf, and mizuna)
1 medium Lebanese cucumber, sliced lengthways
1 celery stick, chopped on the diagonal
1 small green pepper, deseeded and thinly sliced
1 small ripe Hass avocado, halved, stoned and diced
fresh basil leaves, to garnish

Dressing

4 tbsp extra-virgin olive oil
1 tbsp white wine vinegar
freshly ground black pepper
pinch of sugar
1 tsp Dijon mustard

- *Place the dressing ingredients in a screw-top jar and shake well.*
- Toss the green salad in a large salad bowl and pour the dressing over. Garnish with fresh basil.

Carbohydrate content per serving: **6** *grams*

Tomatoes and Mozzarella with mango dressing

For 2   2 large vine-ripened tomatoes, thickly sliced
100 grams Mozzarella, sliced
slices of mango and lime zest, to garnish

Dressing

4 tbsp extra-virgin olive oil
1 tbsp white wine vinegar
2 slices fresh mango, puréed
½ tsp sesame seeds
pinch of rock salt
freshly ground black pepper

- *Place the dressing ingredients in a screw-top jar and shake well.*
- *Place slices of tomato and Mozzarella alternately around the circumference of a plate, and drizzle over the dressing. Garnish with slices of mango and lime zest.*

Carbohydrate content per serving: **5** *grams*

Cucumber and bean sprout salad

For 2   50 grams bean sprouts
1 Lebanese cucumber, sliced lengthways julienne-style
1 yellow pepper, deseeded and very thinly sliced
handful of rocket leaves
2 tbsp chopped fresh chives

Dressing

4 tbsp extra-virgin olive oil
1 tbsp balsamic vinegar
1 tsp Dijon mustard
pinch of granulated sugar
freshly ground black pepper

- *Place the ingredients of the dressing in a screw-top jar and shake well. Toss the salad and drizzle the dressing over. Garnish with chopped chives.*

*Carbohydrate content per serving: **4** grams*

Cucumber and mint soured-cream salad

For 2   1 Lebanese cucumber, diced
3 spring onions, finely chopped
1 garlic clove, peeled and finely chopped
150 ml soured cream
1 tsp freshly squeezed lemon juice
1 tbsp chopped fresh chives
1 tbsp chopped fresh mint
pinch of rock salt
freshly ground black pepper
sprigs of fresh mint and lime zest, to garnish

- *Mix together the ingredients of the salad in a medium bowl, season to taste and chill in the fridge for 1–2 hours. Serve chilled, garnished with sprigs of fresh mint and lime zest.*

Carbohydrate content per serving: **6** *grams*

Rocket and avocado salad

For 2
1 large handful of rocket leaves
1 tbsp chopped fresh basil
1 tbsp chopped fresh coriander
1 ripe Hass avocado, halved, stoned, peeled and
  cubed

Dressing

4 tbsp extra-virgin olive oil
1 tbsp white wine vinegar
½ tsp Dijon mustard
pinch of rock salt
freshly ground black pepper

• *Place the olive oil, white wine vinegar, mustard and seasoning in a screw-top jar and shake thoroughly. Toss the salad, and drizzle the dressing over.*

*Carbohydrate content per serving: **2** grams*

Asparagus and smoked mackerel salad

For 2   6 fresh asparagus spears
1 pak choy, halved lengthways
1 tbsp freshly squeezed lime juice
2 tbsp extra-virgin olive oil
100 grams wild rocket leaves
2 smoked mackerel fillets
150 ml crème fraîche
freshly ground black pepper

- *Wash the asparagus and cook in a pan of boiling water for approximately 4 minutes (or microwave on high for 2–3 minutes).*
- *Set aside to cool.*
- *Cook the pak choy in a microwave on high for approximately 2–3 minutes with 1 tablespoon water.*
- *In a large bowl, mix together the pak choy, asparagus, lime juice and olive oil.*
- *Place a bed of rocket on each plate, and spoon over the pak choy and asparagus mixture.*
- *Top with the smoked mackerel fillets and crème fraîche and season with freshly ground black pepper.*

Carbohydrate content per serving: **10** *grams*

Smoked mackerel and rocket salad

For 2 Guacamole (page 203)
100 grams wild rocket leaves
150 grams smoked mackerel
freshly ground black pepper
fresh lemon

- *Prepare the guacamole.*
- *Top a bed of rocket with guacamole and smoked mackerel.*
- *Season to taste with freshly ground black pepper.*
- *Sprinkle some freshly squeezed lemon juice over the mackerel.*
- *Serve immediately.*

Carbohydrate content per serving: 6 grams

Salad Niçoise

For 2 150 grams tuna tinned in spring water, drained and flaked
2 hard-boiled eggs, peeled and quartered
4 cherry tomatoes, halved
4 leaves of iceberg lettuce, chopped roughly
8 olives, black, green or mixed
100 grams French beans, cooked and chopped

- *Mix together the ingredients and serve immediately with a light dressing.*

Carbohydrate content per serving: 7 grams

Grilled Halloumi salad

For 2
15 black olives, stones removed and halved
15 green olives, stones removed and halved
1 tbsp fresh oregano
1 tbsp chopped fresh basil leaves
1 garlic clove, peeled and grated
1 celery stalk, chopped into small segments
1 tbsp lime juice
2 tbsp extra-virgin olive oil
200 grams Halloumi cheese
freshly ground black pepper
2 tsp linseed oil

- *Mix together the olives, herbs, garlic, celery, lime juice, extra-virgin olive oil, linseed oil and pepper in a bowl and marinate in the fridge.*
- *Slice the Halloumi into 1-cm slices and place on aluminium foil.*
- *Heat under a preheated grill for approximately 1–2 minutes until brown.*
- *Transfer the cheese to plates and top with the marinated olive salad.*
- *Serve immediately.*

*Carbohydrate content per serving: **12** grams*

Avocado and smoked salmon salad

For 2   1 medium Hass avocado, halved, stoned, peeled and
diced
100 grams smoked salmon, sliced
1 tbsp freshly squeezed lemon juice
100 ml crème fraîche
freshly ground black pepper

- *Mix together the avocado and smoked salmon.*
- *Drizzle over the lemon juice and top with crème fraîche.*
- *Season to taste and serve immediately.*

Carbohydrate content per serving: **4** *grams*

Parma ham and rocket salad

For 2   100 grams wild rocket leaves
150 grams Parma ham
50 grams cucumber, sliced into ribbons
75 grams tomato salsa (page 225)

- *Place a bed of rocket on a plate and top with Parma ham, tomato salsa and cucumber ribbons.*

Carbohydrate content per serving: **10** *grams*

Mangetout, French bean and red cabbage salad
For 2   50 grams pine nuts
         25 grams sesame seeds
         150 grams mangetout
         100 grams French beans, topped and sliced
            diagonally
         100 grams red cabbage, finely sliced
         Soya and ginger dressing (page 226)

- *Lightly toast the pine nuts and sesame seeds in a large frying pan for approximately 1–2 minutes.*
- *Place the mangetout, French beans and red cabbage in a microwave-safe dish, and microwave on high for 3 minutes.*
- *Mix together the vegetables, pine nuts and sesame seeds and drizzle over some soya and ginger dressing.*
- *Serve immediately.*

*Carbohydrate content per serving: **9** grams*

Chapter 16

Sauces and dressings

Satay sauce

For 2
- 1 tbsp extra-virgin olive oil
- 1 small red onion, peeled and finely chopped
- 1 garlic clove, peeled and finely chopped
- 1 small red chilli, deseeded and finely chopped
- 3 tbsp peanut butter
- 100 ml coconut cream
- ½ tsp Worcester sauce

- *Heat the extra-virgin olive oil in a small saucepan and sauté the onion, garlic and chilli for 1–2 minutes.*
- *Remove from the heat and stir in the peanut butter, coconut milk and Worcester sauce.*
- *Heat through over a low heat, then allow to cool.*

*Carbohydrate content per serving: **9** grams*

Balsamic vinaigrette

For 2   1 tbsp balsamic vinegar
         4 tbsp extra-virgin olive oil
         half a garlic clove, peeled and chopped finely
         1 slice fresh root ginger, peeled and chopped finely
         freshly ground black pepper

 •   *Place all the ingredients into a screw-top jar and
     shake to mix thoroughly.*

Carbohydrate content per serving: 2 grams

Lime and coriander vinaigrette

For 2   4 tbsp extra-virgin olive oil
1 tbsp white wine vinegar
1 garlic clove, peeled and finely chopped
1 tbsp freshly squeezed lime juice
1 tbsp fresh coriander
freshly ground black pepper

- *Place all the ingredients into a screw-top jar and shake to mix thoroughly.*

*Carbohydrate content per serving: **2** grams*

Basil and pesto sauce

For 2   40 grams chopped fresh basil leaves
          1 garlic clove, peeled and finely chopped
          25 grams pine nuts, lightly toasted
          25 grams Parmesan cheese, freshly grated
          freshly ground black pepper
          45 ml extra-virgin olive oil

- *Put the basil, garlic, pine nuts and Parmesan cheese in a blender. Season to taste then mix.*
- *Gradually add the olive oil while blending to a smooth and even consistency.*

*Carbohydrate content per serving: **2** grams*

Coriander and pesto sauce

For 2   30 grams fresh coriander leaves
1 garlic clove, peeled and chopped
25 grams pine nuts
25 grams grated Parmesan cheese
freshly ground black pepper
45 ml extra-virgin olive oil

- *In a blender, mix the coriander, garlic, pine nuts and Parmesan cheese, adding seasoning to taste.*
- *Continue to blend, adding the olive oil until you get a smooth and even consistency.*

*Carbohydrate content per serving: **2** grams*

Horseradish sauce

For 4   100 ml crème fraîche
1 tbsp freshly grated horseradish
½ tsp caster sugar
1 tbsp white wine vinegar
freshly ground black pepper

- Mix the ingredients in a blender, then chill in the fridge for 4 hours.

Carbohydrate content per serving: **5** *grams*

French vinaigrette

For 2   4 tbsp extra-virgin olive oil
1 tbsp white wine vinegar
½ tsp mustard powder
half a garlic clove, peeled and finely chopped
freshly ground black pepper

- Place all the ingredients into a screw-top jar and shake to mix well.

*Carbohydrate content per serving: **1** gram*

. . . .

Tomato salsa

For 2   4 large vine-ripened tomatoes, deseeded and finely chopped
2 medium shallots, peeled and diced
1 garlic clove, peeled and grated
1 red chilli, deseeded and finely chopped
1 tbsp chopped fresh basil leaves
1 tbsp chopped fresh marjoram
1 tbsp extra-virgin olive oil

- *Mix the ingredients in a medium bowl, cover and chill for 1 hour.*

*Carbohydrate content per serving: **8** grams*

Soya and ginger dressing

For 2   4 tbsp extra-virgin olive oil
        1 tbsp white wine vinegar
        3–4 drops sesame oil
        ½ tsp fresh ginger, peeled and finely grated
        2 tsp soy sauce

- *Put the ingredients in a screw-top jar and shake to mix well.*

Carbohydrate content per serving: 2 grams

PART III

Weight-Maintenance Phase Recipes

Congratulations! You have achieved the weight loss and it is now time to enjoy yourself a little more. We can now begin to reintroduce higher GI recipes that you can bring into all of the main meals of the day, in moderation and not gain weight. Remember, if you start to gain weight then you are eating too much of these high-GI recipes.

And remember to count! One of the problems of the weight-maintenance phase is that you have to keep your carbohydrate content to within 60–80 grams per day. This is very easy to achieve even though the recipes have a far higher GI content. But remember to count while you are including these recipes. Too many of the weight-maintenance recipes in any one day will definitely break the programme.

So let's begin . . .

Chapter 17 Breakfast

Mango and melon smoothie

For 2   150 grams melon, chopped
½ mango, peeled, stone removed and chopped
250 ml natural yoghurt

- *Purée the fruit until smooth in a blender.*
- *Add the yoghurt and blend with the fruit.*
- *Serve immediately.*

*Carbohydrate content per serving: **24** grams*

Kiwi fruit smoothie

For 2   3 kiwi fruit, peeled and chopped
100 grams raspberries
250 ml natural yoghurt

- *Place the kiwi fruit and raspberries in a blender.*
- *Add the yoghurt and blend until smooth.*
- *Serve immediately.*

*Carbohydrate content per serving: **20** grams*

Fruit platter

For 2   1 medium Seville orange, peeled and divided into
         segments
         ½ mango, peeled and sliced
         50 grams blueberries
         50 grams raspberries
         100 grams grapes
         2 kiwi fruit, peeled and sliced
         100 grams natural yoghurt (optional)

- *Arrange the fruit in a bowl, topped with yoghurt if desired.*
- *Serve immediately.*

*Carbohydrate content per serving: **40** grams*

Whipped cream cheese with fruit

For 2   150 grams whipped cream cheese
         2 kiwi fruit, peeled and sliced
         1 pear, peeled, stone removed and sliced
         75 grams blueberries
         1 tbsp grated almonds

- *Mix together the whipped cream cheese, kiwi fruit, pear and blueberries.*
- *Serve immediately, topped with grated almonds.*

*Carbohydrate content per serving: **27** grams*

Blueberries with mixed nuts and yoghurt

For 2   200 grams blueberries
         50 grams mixed hazelnuts, Brazil nuts and pine nuts,
            chopped
         1 dessertspoon sunflower seeds
         150 grams natural yoghurt

- *Mix together the berries, nuts and seeds.*
- *Top with natural yoghurt and serve immediately.*

*Carbohydrate content per serving: **19** grams*

. . . .

Fruit kebabs

For 2   half a mango, peeled, stone removed and chopped
            into 3-cm cubes
         8 strawberries, halved
         2 kiwi fruit, peeled and chopped into segments
         2 tbsp freshly squeezed lemon juice
         1 tsp runny honey
         100 grams natural yoghurt

- Thread the fruits alternately onto skewers.
- Drizzle over the lemon juice and runny honey.
- Place under a medium grill (no closer than
  approximately 8 cm) for 8–10 minutes, turning once.
- Serve immediately with the natural yoghurt.

*Carbohydrate content per serving: **31** grams*

Peaches and hazelnuts with fromage frais

For 2   200 grams tinned peaches in natural juice
200 grams fromage frais
25 grams hazelnuts, chopped

- *Drain the peaches.*
- *Slice the fruit and mix with the fromage frais.*
- *Gently toast the hazelnuts in a frying pan.*
- *Top the fruit mixture with the toasted hazelnuts and serve immediately.*

*Carbohydrate content per serving: **14** grams*

Pomegranate fruit salad

For 2   1 pomegranate
2 kiwi fruit
1 pomelo
natural yoghurt

- *Cut the pomegranate in half and scrape out the seeds into a medium mixing bowl.*
- *Peel the kiwi fruit and slice finely. Add the slices to the mixing bowl.*
- *Remove the outer skin and the pith from the pomelo and add the segments to the salad.*
- *Mix the fruits together, top with natural yoghurt and serve immediately.*

*Carbohydrate content per serving: **20** grams*

Caponata

For 2
1 large aubergine, chopped and cubed
rock salt
2 tbsp extra-virgin olive oil
1 onion, peeled and diced
1 garlic clove, peeled and finely chopped
1 medium red pepper, deseeded and sliced
1 medium green pepper, deseeded and sliced
1 celery stick, chopped into 2–3-cm segments
1 courgette, chopped diagonally into large pieces
10 cherry tomatoes, peeled and chopped
1 tbsp chopped fresh chives
1 tbsp chopped fresh basil leaves
1 tbsp chopped fresh flat-leaf parsley
1 tsp brown sugar
50 ml white wine vinegar
10 green olives, pitted and halved
freshly ground black pepper
fresh parsley leaves, to garnish

- *Place the aubergine cubes in a colander, sprinkle with salt and leave for 20–30 minutes, then rinse with cold water and pat dry.*
- *Heat the extra-virgin olive oil in a medium frying pan and sauté the onion and garlic for 2 minutes.*
- *Add the peppers and celery and cook for a further 2 minutes, then add the aubergine and courgette.*
- *Cook on a low heat for 3–4 minutes. Add the tomatoes and gently simmer for about 10–12 minutes.*

- *Add the herbs, sugar, white wine vinegar and olives.*
- *Season to taste and gently simmer for a further 5 minutes. Garnish with chopped fresh parsley leaves.*

*Carbohydrate content per serving: **20** grams*

Roasted vegetables with fusilli

For 2   1 medium aubergine, sliced thinly
1 large courgette, sliced
2 shallots, peeled and sliced
1 red pepper, deseeded and sliced
1 yellow pepper, deseeded and sliced
1 garlic clove, peeled and finely chopped
2 slices fresh ginger, peeled and finely chopped
1–2 tbsp extra-virgin olive oil
freshly ground black pepper
60 grams fusilli
2 tbsp fresh basil leaves, chopped
fresh flat-leaf parsley, to garnish

- *Place the aubergine, courgette, shallots, peppers, ginger and garlic in a large roasting tin. Drizzle over the extra-virgin olive oil and season to taste.*
- *Roast the vegetables in a preheated oven at 200 degrees C (gas mark 6) for 25–30 minutes, until slightly charred.*
- *Cook the fusilli until al dente then drain.*
- *Combine the pasta and the vegetables in a large mixing bowl, stir in the basil and serve immediately, garnished with flesh flat-leaf parsley.*

Carbohydrate content per serving: **31** *grams*

Emmental and pancetta pasta

For 2   80 grams penne pasta
150 grams broccoli florets
4 rashers pancetta
100 grams Emmental cheese, grated
100 ml crème fraîche
freshly ground black pepper
1 tbsp chopped fresh chives

- *Cook the pasta in a large pan of boiling salted water for approximately 8–10 minutes.*

At the same time

- *Microwave the broccoli florets for approximately 2 minutes. Grill the bacon for 1–2 minutes until crispy, then chop.*
- *Drain the pasta. Stir in the broccoli, Emmental, pancetta and crème fraîche.*
- *Transfer the mixture to a heat-proof serving dish and place under a medium grill for about 1 minute.*
- *Serve immediately, seasoned with black pepper and garnished with chopped chives.*

Carbohydrate content per serving: **30** *grams*

Angel hair pasta with mozzarella

For 2
80 grams angel hair pasta
150 grams mangetout, trimmed and sliced
100 grams plum tomatoes, halved
1 medium garlic clove, peeled and chopped finely
1 tbsp freshly squeezed lime juice
2 tbsp extra-virgin olive oil
100 grams mozzarella cheese, sliced
freshly ground black pepper

- *Cook the pasta in a saucepan of boiling salted water for 8–10 minutes.*
- *Add the mangetout to the pan after 6 minutes.*
- *Drain the pasta, mix in the tomatoes and garlic, lime juice and olive oil.*
- *Top with mozzarella cheese and place under a medium grill (no closer than 8–10 cm) for approximately 1 minute (or until the cheese starts to brown).*
- *Serve immediately, seasoned with freshly ground black pepper.*

*Carbohydrate content per serving: **35** grams*

Tiger prawns with tagliatelle

For 2
80 grams tagliatelle
2 tbsp extra-virgin olive oil
10 large cooked tiger prawns, peeled
10 cherry tomatoes, halved
100 grams spinach leaves
freshly ground black pepper

- *Cook the tagliatelle for 8–10 minutes in a large pan of salted water.*
- *Just before the pasta is ready, heat the extra-virgin olive oil in a wok and stir-fry the prawns, tomatoes and spinach for 2 minutes.*
- *Serve the pasta topped with the prawn and tomato mixture, and season to taste with freshly ground black pepper.*

Carbohydrate content per serving: **35** *grams*

Pappardelle with crab

For 2   60 grams pappardelle, dry or fresh
2 tbsp extra-virgin olive oil
1 garlic clove, peeled and diced
2 slices of fresh ginger, peeled and diced
250 grams fresh white crab meat
150 grams mixed wild rocket and spinach leaves
1 tbsp chopped fresh coriander leaves
1 tbsp chopped fresh basil leaves
freshly ground black pepper

- Cook the pappardelle until *al dente*.

At the same time
- *Heat the extra-virgin olive oil in a medium frying pan.*
- *Sauté the garlic and ginger for 1–2 minutes, then stir in the crab meat.*
- *Stir in the rocket and spinach leaves and heat for 1–2 minutes.*
- *Drain the pasta.*
- *Stir in the crab mixture, adding the coriander and basil.*
- *Season to taste and serve immediately.*

*Carbohydrate content per serving: **23** grams*

Fettuccine with pancetta

For 2   80 grams fettuccine, dry or fresh
2 tbsp extra-virgin olive oil
6 slices pancetta, chopped into large pieces
1 medium leek, trimmed and sliced lengthways
150 grams baby spinach leaves
100 grams mascarpone cheese
30 grams freshly grated Parmesan cheese
freshly ground black pepper

- *Place the fettuccine in a large pan of boiling water and cook for about 8 minutes (or 3–4 minutes for fresh pasta).*
- *Heat the olive oil in a medium frying pan and cook the pancetta for 2–3 minutes.*
- *Add the leek and spinach and stir-fry for a further 3–4 minutes.*
- *Stir in the mascarpone and warm gently for 2–3 minutes.*
- *Drain the pasta and stir in the pancetta mixture. Sprinkle over some Parmesan cheese, season to taste and serve immediately.*

*Carbohydrate content per serving: **32** grams*

Chapter **19** Dinner

Salmon fettuccine carbonara

For 2
1 fresh salmon steak (approximately 150 grams)
1 tbsp extra-virgin olive oil
60 grams dried fettuccine
100 ml double cream
50 grams freshly grated Parmesan cheese
freshly ground black pepper
1 tbsp chopped fresh chives

- Brush the salmon steak with the extra-virgin olive oil.
- Grill the salmon for about 5 minutes under a medium grill, turning once.
- Remove the salmon and allow to cool, then flake the flesh, discarding all bones and skin.

At the same time

- *Cook the fettuccine until al dente.*
- *Whisk the cream.*
- *Drain the fettuccine and transfer to a large mixing bowl.*
- *Stir in the flaked salmon, cream and grated Parmesan.*
- *Season to taste with pepper and garnish with chopped fresh chives.*
- *Serve immediately.*

*Carbohydrate content per serving: **22** grams*

Nasi Goreng

For 2   60 grams Arborio rice
25 grams unsalted butter
2 large free-range eggs, beaten
2 tbsp extra-virgin olive oil
1 medium red onion, peeled and diced
1 garlic clove, peeled and chopped
2 slices of fresh ginger, peeled and finely chopped
1 medium red chilli, deseeded and finely sliced
1 medium orange pepper, deseeded and finely sliced
1 medium yellow pepper, deseeded and finely sliced
2 spring onions, chopped diagonally into 3-cm
    lengths
1 tbsp chopped fresh coriander leaves
1 tbsp chopped fresh marjoram leaves
1 tbsp soy sauce
freshly ground black pepper
100 grams fresh baby spinach leaves

- *Cook the rice.*

At the same time
- *Heat the butter in a medium pan and scramble the eggs with the marjoram and coriander, stirring constantly. Cover and set aside.*
- *Heat the extra-virgin olive oil in a wok and stir-fry the onion, garlic, ginger, chilli, peppers and spring onions for 2–3 minutes.*
- *Stir in the scrambled eggs, cooked rice and soy sauce and stir-fry for a further 2 minutes, seasoning to taste.*
- *Arrange a bed of spinach on the plates and top with the nasi goreng.*

Carbohydrate content per serving: **27** *grams*

Lasagne with Bolognese sauce

For 4   2 tbsp extra-virgin olive oil
1 medium red onion, peeled and diced
2 garlic cloves, peeled and chopped
200 grams lean beef mince (or vegetarian substitute)
1 tbsp tomato purée
150 ml chicken stock
1 tbsp chopped fresh basil leaves
freshly ground black pepper
25 grams unsalted butter
30 grams plain flour
150 ml milk
4 sheets dried lasagne
1 tbsp freshly grated Parmesan cheese
100 grams spinach leaves

- *Heat the extra-virgin olive oil in a medium frying pan, and sauté the onion and garlic for 2–3 minutes.*
- *Add the mince and stir until browned.*
- *Stir in the tomato purée, chicken stock and basil, season to taste and simmer gently for 3–4 minutes.*

At the same time
- *Melt the butter in a saucepan and remove from the heat. Stir in the flour until the mixture is smooth.*
- *Return the pan to a gentle heat and gradually add the milk, stirring constantly, until the sauce just begins to thicken.*
- *Remove from the heat, continuing to stir.*
- *Spread about a quarter of the Bolognese sauce on the base of a medium roasting tin, top with white sauce and cover with a sheet of lasagne.*
- *Repeat this three times in layers, then cover with the*

*final sheet of lasagne, pour on the remaining white
sauce and sprinkle with grated Parmesan cheese.*
- *Cook in the centre of a preheated over at 180 degrees
C (gas mark 4) for approximately 25–30 minutes.*
- *Divide the lasagne into 4 equal portions, season to
taste and serve with fresh spinach leaves.*

Carbohydrate content per serving: **20** grams

• •

Spaghetti Bolognese

For 2   2 tbsp extra-virgin olive oil
1 medium red onion, peeled and diced
2 garlic cloves, peeled and chopped
250 grams turkey mince
1 tbsp tomato purée
150 ml chicken stock
1 tbsp chopped fresh basil leaves
freshly ground black pepper
60 grams wholemeal spaghetti

- Heat the extra-virgin olive oil in a medium frying pan,
and sauté the onion and garlic for 2–3 minutes.
- Add the turkey mince and brown.
- Stir in the tomato purée, chicken stock and basil,
season to taste and simmer gently for 3–4 minutes.

At the same time
- *Cook the spaghetti until al dente.*
- *Drain the spaghetti and mix in the Bolognese sauce.*
- *Season to taste and serve immediately.*

Carbohydrate content per serving: **27** grams

Turkey steaks with basil and tomato bulgar

For 2   150 grams fresh plum tomatoes
1 medium red onion, peeled and diced
2 tbsp extra-virgin olive oil
1 garlic clove, peeled and finely chopped
30 grams bulgar wheat
50 ml chicken stock
4 medium turkey steaks, approximately 100 grams
   each
a little butter
1 tbsp chopped fresh basil leaves
freshly ground black pepper

- *To peel the tomatoes, make a shallow cross in the skin at the base.*
- *Place the tomatoes in a bowl of boiling water for about 30 seconds, then drain off the water.*
- *Immerse the tomatoes in cold water for a few seconds and the skin will peel off relatively easily. Then chop the tomatoes.*
- *Sauté the onion in the olive oil. Stir in the garlic.*
- *Stir in the bulgar wheat and the chopped tomatoes.*
- *Add the chicken stock, bring to the boil and simmer for about 10 minutes.*
- *Remove from the heat and allow to settle for approximately 10 minutes.*

At the same time
- *Place the turkey steaks in an ovenproof dish, dot with butter, cover with pierced aluminium foil and cook in a preheated oven at 180 degrees C (gas mark 4) for approximately 15 minutes.*
- *Serve the turkey steaks with the chopped basil and bulgar wheat and season to taste.*

*Carbohydrate content per serving: **18** grams*

Chicken escalopes with puréed peas

For 2   2 chicken breasts, skin removed
2 tbsp plain flour, seasoned
100 grams fresh peas
100 grams tinned chickpeas, drained and rinsed
1 tbsp chopped fresh parsley leaves
freshly ground black pepper
sprigs of fresh flat-leaf parsley, to garnish

- *Place the chicken between two pieces of clingfilm and flatten with a rolling pin to a thickness of about 10 mm.*
- *Remove the chicken from the clingfilm and toss in seasoned flour.*
- *Cook under a preheated grill (no closer than 10 cm) for 3–4 minutes per side.*

At the same time
- *Cook the peas in boiling, salted water for 3–4 minutes.*
- *Add the chickpeas and cook for a further 1–2 minutes.*
- *Drain the peas, add the chopped parsley, then blend until smooth.*
- *Serve the puréed peas with the chicken, and season to taste.*
- *Garnish with fresh flat-leaf parsley.*

Carbohydrate content per serving: **27** *grams*

PART IV

Health and Exercise

In this part of the book, we start by addressing the health-giving benefits of the New Protein Diet and explaining some of the technical aspects. But this is only part of the story. Every diet book should have a chapter devoted to exercise – because even a moderate amount of regular exercise produces immense benefits for our general health – but this programme is probably going to be very different from any other you have encountered. It's not going to involve weights, complicated aerobic exercises, any special equipment, or even require much time in your busy schedule.

Chapter **20** Eating for health

Healthy eating implies boring, tasteless food: salad (again) without vinaigrette, plain vegetables, and fat-free (therefore taste-free) meals. This chapter will completely destroy this myth, demonstrating that delicious food can also be healthy. It will explain why this diet is made up the way it is, why certain foods are included and others are excluded: in essence, why it works, and why you can't break the rules and still be successful. If you take the time to read this chapter (and re-read it later), you will understand what you have to do – and why – and you will start to take control of your own health. That is the whole point of the book. It is not just to lose weight (as fat), but also to be fitter and healthier, feel better, have more self-confidence, and enjoy your life so much more. While losing your fat, you will achieve all these other goals without even trying. But you will find it much easier to stick to the programme if you understand how it works, rather than just following it blindly.

In Chapter 1, I briefly discussed the major essential components in our diet: proteins, fats, carbohydrates, vitamins and minerals. Here I will elaborate on the essential functions of each of these food groups, focusing a little bit on their main actions in keeping us healthy, how we can burn our body fat by altering the various proportions of these groups in the diet, and at the same time not only maintain our health but actually improve it.

During this diet, no one will feel hungry or deprived – apart, perhaps, from totally addicted chocaholics, and even they can return to a decreased level of addiction after they have lost most of their unwanted kilos.

Proteins

These are the building blocks of the body. Or, to be more accurate, proteins are made up of amino acids, which are the building blocks of the body. Every protein is constructed of many amino acids, and when we eat foods containing protein, our digestive system breaks down the protein into its component amino acids, and our body then joins them together again as the structural proteins we need, a little like a human Lego set.

Amino acids – the building blocks of life

Proteins are essential for building not only the structures we can see – like skin, bones, hair and nails – but also all the myriad tissues we can't see but which keep us alive, like the blood cells, immune system, nervous system and chemicals that make reactions occur, called enzymes. The bottom line is, we need certain proteins for life.

Although all of the proteins we require can be supplied from plant sources, 'complete' proteins (which means they contain all of the essential amino acids we need) come primarily from animal sources: beef, pork, fish, poultry and eggs. So animal sources of protein will form the basis of this diet for two main reasons: firstly, they will supply all of the essential amino acids to prevent protein deficiencies (which are very serious), and secondly, it is much more complicated to ensure that you obtain all of the necessary amino acids from plants, especially for the beginner.

To make things even easier, animal proteins (beef, pork, fish, poultry and eggs) have negligible amounts of carbohydrates, so they switch off the insulin mechanism and switch on the fat-burning system. But what about the fat, and calories, in these foods? Fats will be discussed in the next section, but suffice it to say that if you switch off the fat-storage mechanism, the fats you eat in your diet will not be deposited as fat in your body. In the same way, if you switch off the fat-storage mechanism, the calorie content of foods is irrelevant – so ignore it. When you have switched on the fat-burning mechanism, it doesn't matter how many calories you eat, you will not put on weight, and you will lose fat – medically.

Fats

Contrary to popular belief, all fats are *not* bad for you. Some are, but probably not the ones you expect. Let's put the fat myth into perspective. We need certain fats for life. Hard though it may be to accept – especially after years of indoctrination – I'm afraid it's not only untrue that all fat in the diet is bad for you, it's positively wrong. We need fats for many reasons: to build cell walls, construct sheaths around nerve cells, and form hormones (chemical messengers in the body), to name just a few essential roles of fats in the body.

Like proteins, fats are made up of their own building blocks (called fatty acids), and we need certain essential fatty acids to live. We also need some fat in our diet for the correct absorption of essential components of the diet. For example, some of the vitamins we need are *fat soluble*, which means they 'dissolve' in fats but not in water. No fat, no absorption of certain essential vitamins (this will be discussed in more detail later).

But all fats are not equal. Some are very good, some not so good. Essential fatty acids are usually divided into two groups: omega-3 and omega-6.

- Omega-3 fatty acids are found in oily fish (such as herring, mackerel, salmon, sardines and tuna), fish oils, egg yolks, nuts, nut oils, and certain vegetable oils (especially flaxseed).
- Omega-6 fatty acids are found in egg yolks, seeds and seed oils (in particular sunflower, safflower and sesame), whole grains, certain vegetables and vegetable oils. Omega-6 fatty acids are also present in evening primrose and borage oils.

A special mention must be made of olive oil, which has a high proportion of monounsaturated oils. Although it is not rich in *essential* fatty acids, it is incredibly healthy, not least because of its vitamin E, magnesium, and antioxidant content – especially polyphenols.

So, obviously, we are going to incorporate these fats into our diet. But we are not going to *add* them to the diet, we are going to *replace* certain of the other types of fat in the diet with these 'healthy' fats. For example, by cooking with olive oil, and eating fish, eggs and certain vegetables, we create a diet high in protein, essential fatty acids, vitamins, minerals, and antioxidants (more about these later), and yet with no refined carbohydrates. Simple!

But what about the fats? A large egg alone provides about 100 kilocalories! This must lead to fat deposition around our midriff, among other places, mustn't it?

Wrong again!

You will not gain weight (as fat) on this diet. You may increase your body protein (as muscle, which is obviously good for you), but you will still lose body fat. How can this be? Surely if you eat more calories than you need, you must gain weight? No, this is the fallacy of the calorie-control diet theory. As I briefly explained back in Chapter 1, the body is not a simple combustion engine. It functions by a very complex system of interactions, and if you switch off the fat-storage system (by reducing carbohydrates below a particular level), it will burn body fat even if you are eating more calories than you absolutely require – provided the extra calories are not carbohydrates. Extra fat intake when the body is in fat-burning mode is simply passed out of the body again (mostly in the urine), without being absorbed, and without being stored as fat. So you can see that provided you switch off the fat-storage mechanism, you can eat more fats without gaining weight.

I can easily prove the fallacy of the calorie-counting system of dieting. Some people have a medical condition that leads to problems with the absorption of certain foods from the intestine. No matter how much they eat of those foods, none are absorbed into the body, and the patient gradually loses weight (and health) despite a high-calorie intake.

Basic fallacy of low-calorie diets

High calorie intake

Absorbs food normally

Gains weight

Poor absorption of food

Losing weight – despite high calorie intake – because *food not absorbed by body*

According to the calorie-counting theory of dieting, this high-calorie intake should mean that these patients gain weight. On the contrary, due to their inability to absorb food, they lose weight. The obvious conclusion from this evidence is that making decisions on health without taking into account the complex interactions that occur within the human body will inevitably result in major errors of judgement. The concept that simply restricting calories will cause fat loss is one such error. *The 95 per cent failure rate of this method proves it does not work.*

So by activating the fat-burning mechanism in the body, you will lose your body fat, even if you are ingesting more calories as fat or protein. And because you are eating the 'right' food, you will be healthier, fitter and slimmer.

Do not misinterpret the message of this chapter. It is not intended to advocate a high-fat diet. Although you are eating 'pure' fats, you will actually be eating *less* fat, because most of the 'bad' fats are incorporated in foods with refined sugars and carbohydrates (such as cakes, pastries, pizza, pies, processed and packaged foods, fast foods, crisps and chips), which you have excluded from your diet. Instead, you have replaced them with essential fatty acids in eggs, fish, vegetables and nuts, among others.

These foods are more than just 'fats', even 'essential fats'. They contain high-quality complete proteins, essential vitamins and minerals, and are major sources of antioxidants, which basically keep us healthy, prevent cancer and various other unpleasant medical conditions, and seriously help to prevent ageing. So before we complain about the dangerous aspects of these fats (and there is a considerable amount of controversy about exactly how dangerous certain fats in the diet are, with strong evidence to suggest that the 'all saturated fats are bad' theory has major flaws), let us also remember the considerable benefits that some very good fats provide for our health and well-being.

Carbohydrates

These provide energy, and little else. 'Refined' carbohydrates provide energy, and *nothing* else, apart from causing the increased production of insulin, which promotes fat storage and prevents the burning of body fat. It would seem fairly obvious to the most casual observer that we don't need refined carbohydrates in our lives, and therefore we are going to exclude them from our diets.

However, apart from refined sugar, carbohydrates are seldom 'pure', but rather mixed with other constituents in various foods. These can be in foods, also containing fats, that are bad for your health (for example chips, cakes, pizzas and so forth), or in foods that are good for you, such as vegetables. The carbohydrates in fresh vegetables are very different from those in refined foods. Fresh vegetables contain what are known as 'complex' carbohydrates, which means they are absorbed much more slowly and more evenly over a period of time, as opposed to the rapid absorption (and associated rapid release of insulin) which occurs with refined sugars. Of much more importance with regard to health, carbohydrates in fresh vegetables are incorporated with vitamins, minerals, proteins and fibre – all of which we need for survival. They are not associated with refined fats, only essential fatty acids (in some vegetables).

I hope you can see the pattern of healthy dieting emerging. It is not about avoiding all fats and eating smaller amounts of food to lower the calorie intake. This results in failed diets in 95 per cent of cases. Successful dieting – to lose fat not protein – involves reducing carbohydrate intake in the form of 'bad' carbohydrates, to literally switch on our intrinsic fat-burning mechanism.

Vitamins and minerals

The simplest way of explaining vitamins and minerals is that they are substances that we require in small quantities in our diet.

Absolutely essential for well-being, they *must* feature in a healthy, weight-loss diet. Happily, they will be included naturally if you select the correct balance of foods. Vitamins and minerals are necessary to facilitate certain chemical reactions in our cells, and some (such as vitamins A, C and E and the mineral selenium) also function as antioxidants, which help to prevent diseases and ageing by mopping up what are known as 'free radicals'. But what exactly are antioxidants and free radicals?

In each individual cell in your body (of which you have trillions) there are thousands of chemical reactions occurring every second. To release the energy from food, these chemical reactions produce 'free radicals', which are essentially molecules that have lost an electron.

Free radical formation

Molecule → Losing electron → Free radical

Their natural reaction is to try to take an electron from another molecule, which will cause damage to the cells in your body – especially as this is occurring millions of times per second.

Free radical → Free radical 'steals' → New free radical
electron from formed
another molecule

This is not good, as it sets off chain reactions of 'stealing' electrons, which weaken your cellular defences against disease and infection. Obviously, you need to stop the process by 'wiping up' the free radicals before they can cause any damage.

This is where antioxidants come into the picture, our knights in shining armour! Antioxidants mop up the free radicals, preventing damage (and long-term disease), keeping us healthy, and delaying the ageing process. They are the closest we have come to the elixir of life in over one million years of existence.

Where do these wondrous things come from? Antioxidants occur in two main forms: as naturally occurring proteins in the body (which we make from essential proteins in our diet), and as various constituents in our diet that are necessary for the proteins to do their job effectively. These 'various constituents' are essential fatty acids (from eggs, oily fish and certain vegetable oils), and vitamins and minerals (from beef, pork, lamb, poultry, fish, shellfish, fresh fruit and vegetables, and dairy produce).

All of the essential vitamins and minerals we need are supplied in dairy produce, fresh vegetables, and animal foods (beef, pork, lamb, fish, poultry, eggs). And as several of the vitamins are *fat soluble* (vitamins A, D, E and K), we need a certain amount of fat in the diet for their effective absorption.

Now where have you seen this particular list of foods before?

Part I has provided guidelines for implementing the principles of the diet (and Part II featured lots of delicious recipes that will enable you to put the diet into practice), but now you can see that if you eat the correct foods, in the correct proportions, you will lose fat naturally and without hunger, become much healthier, and at the same time increase your protection against disease and ageing. And all this will cost little or no more than you spend on food at the moment, and take no more time out of your day. Now you will begin to appreciate that what seemed too good to be true at the start of the book actually makes sense. And for the first time on any diet you understand what you are doing, and you are in control.

A nutritionally safe diet

A responsible diet should allow you to lose weight easily and eat healthily at the same time. This diet does just that. You may be cutting out refined carbohydrates, but you will be receiving all the nutrients you need for your well-being from other food sources, as follows:

- *Essential amino acids.* These are provided by the proteins in animal products: meat, fish poultry, shellfish, eggs and dairy produce. While plants certainly have proteins, the only plant source with *complete* proteins is soya (and its derivatives). By contrast, all animal products have complete proteins (see page 250).
- *Omega-3 fatty acids.* Most prevalent in oily fish such as salmon, mackerel, herrings, sardines and tuna, omega-3 fatty acids can also be obtained from egg yolks, as well as nuts and certain seeds (e.g. flaxseed oil).
- *Omega-6 fatty acids.* These are most prevalent in egg yolks, seeds (particularly sunflower, safflower and sesame), whole grains and some vegetables.
- *Vitamin A.* Typical foods with high concentrations of vitamin A are fish, egg yolk, butter, cheese, carrots, red peppers, spinach, tomatoes, and mangetout. This vitamin is present in most fruits and vegetables, but in varying proportions.
- *Vitamin B_1 (thiamin).* Excellent sources in this diet are pork, fresh fish (especially salmon), certain nuts (cashews, Brazils, peanuts, pine nuts) and sesame seeds.
- *Vitamin B_2 (riboflavin).* This is present in dairy products (cream and cheese), liver, beef, chicken, eggs, fish, shellfish, mushrooms, avocado and almonds.
- *Vitamin B_3 (niacin).* High concentrations are found in fish (especially salmon and tuna), meat, chicken, liver and eggs.

- *Vitamin B₆ (pyridoxine).* This is present in fish (especially tuna), meat (particularly pork), liver, chicken, avocados, nuts (especially walnuts and cashews), tomatoes and tomato purée.
- *Vitamin B₁₂ (cyanocobalamin).* This is the only vitamin *not* found in foods of plant origin. It is present in highest concentrations in liver, seafood, fish (especially sardines, salmon and tuna) and eggs, and in lesser amounts in milk products and meats. Vegetarians are therefore recommended to take a vitamin supplement.
- *Folate.* The highest concentration of folate occurs in liver, but there are also good concentrations in most vegetables (especially green vegetables), meat, poultry, fish, shellfish, eggs and nuts (particularly peanuts and cashews).
- *Vitamin C.* Apart from liver and kidney, vitamin C is not present in animal products and has to be obtained from vegetables (especially red and green peppers, mangetout, tomato, and broccoli) and fruit (strawberries and citrus fruits).
- *Vitamin D.* Oily fish provide by far the highest levels of vitamin D compared with any other food group; mackerel, herring, salmon and, to a much lesser degree, tuna are particularly rich. There is a small amount of vitamin D in eggs and butter.
- *Vitamin E.* The dietary requirements for this vitamin are provided in the diet by nuts (almonds, hazelnuts, peanuts), olives, tomato purée, avocado and fish.
- *Vitamin K.* The best dietary source is undoubtedly green vegetables, such as broccoli, cabbage, lettuce, spring onions and spinach.
- *Selenium.* This mineral is vital for the production of enzymes, and is available in onions, tomatoes, broccoli, bean sprouts and fish.

- *Iron.* You will obtain sufficient amounts of this important mineral from fish, nuts, liver, meat, chicken, sesame seeds and green vegetables.
- *Manganese.* This is found in eggs, nuts and green vegetables.
- *Copper.* Nuts, mushrooms and green vegetables are all good sources of copper.
- *Zinc.* Excellent sources include eggs, sesame seeds, nuts (especially cashew nuts and almonds), herbs and many vegetables.
- *Potassium.* This is abundant in fish, herbs, garlic, onion, vegetables, mushrooms and citrus fruit.
- *Calcium.* Important for the manufacture of bones, this is found in dairy products, fish, green vegetables (especially broccoli and parsley) and herbs.
- *Sulphur.* You can obtain this from garlic, onions, fish, eggs, nuts, cabbage and meat.

Don't worry, you don't need to learn any of the details in the above list of nutrients. I have merely included it to show you, in a very simplistic way, that you are receiving all that you require for good health by following this diet, which allows unrestricted consumption of these essential nutrients, in the form of delicious meals. The recipes in Part II have been carefully devised to help you receive a nutritionally balanced diet; for more ideas on how to balance your meals, turn to the menu plans on pages 57–61.

Chapter 21 Why exercise?

Do you *have* to exercise when you are on this diet? The answer is no, you don't *have* to exercise, because you *will* lose body fat on this diet without exercise, and you won't lose much fat from exercise alone unless you exercise for long periods every day – which has the double disadvantage of stimulating hunger (so you need to eat more food) and also stimulating the production of more insulin, which then converts the extra food into fat! Now you begin to understand why it is very difficult to lose weight by exercise alone and how it is virtually impossible to exercise on a low-calorie diet. However, you don't need to do much exercise to achieve *dramatic* changes in your physical appearance when exercise is taken in association with a diet that specifically removes body fat and leaves body musculature intact.

If you really don't want to do any exercise, I have to be honest and say that you don't have to exercise if you only want to lose fat. In other words, you will lose fat and be much slimmer on this diet without specific exercise routines. So if you really are opposed to exercise, read no further.

But with just a little time (less than 15 minutes per day) devoted to easy exercises – which almost *anyone* can do, no matter how out of condition or overweight – you can improve the *shape* of your body and look much more attractive. To understand how you can change the shape of your body in this way, I have to explain a little about anatomy – or the structural make-up of the body – in simple terms. I keep repeating that most of medicine is essentially applied common sense, and you will soon realise how true this is.

The body has an underlying framework made up of bone – the skeleton. This is the scaffolding that supports us. Over the skeleton is a layer of muscle, then a layer of fat and finally the outer covering of skin. So you can easily appreciate that if you reduce the fat layer, you will become slimmer, but if you also – even slightly – tighten or tone-up the muscle layer, you will *suddenly assume a smooth, toned body shape*.

Rather than just being thinner, you will be slimmer *with shape* as a result of the increased muscle tone.

Achieving this attractive body shape does not need to involve complex weight training or exhausting, prolonged aerobic exercises, but rather *a simple series of specially designed exercises which you can perform in the privacy of your own home without expensive equipment*.

Let us return to the primary reason, apart from your health, for being on a diet – simply because, like most people, you want to look better, slimmer and more attractive. And if you succeed, you assume – probably correctly – that you will have more self-confidence. So, surely, if you lose fat you'll look better, feel better and probably have elevated self-esteem and therefore self-confidence. You might think, why bother exercising? It all comes back to the body shape to which you aspire. By that I don't want to give any false impression that I can transform you into a supermodel, but with just a *little* exercising to improve the *tone* of your body, you will reveal the contoured shape of the real you. And it is much better than you think! We can't change our inherent genetic characteristics, but we can definitely change the amount of fat we are carrying around with us. If your muscles are flabby (and they probably are), without exercise you will be slimmer but still a little shapeless.

If, however, you perform 10–15 minutes per day of *very* light exercise – and I mean *very* light – which can be done in your own home at any time of day (without embarrassment) – you will quickly tone up your muscles, and as the fat drops away, you will be left with a much more attractive body shape – with very little effort!

The ultimate underlying purpose of this book is really to demonstrate that you *can* lose your excess fat, tone up your muscles, look great and feel great with *no pain and very little effort.* You will look and feel much better on this integrated programme *within 2 weeks,* although obviously it will take some time to lose all the excess fat at 1–1½ kilos per week, depending on how much there is to lose. All those years of struggling to lose weight are over!

The other major importance of exercise is that it improves circulation. Even a little exercise opens the tiny blood vessels, called capillaries, in all the tissues of the body, so the tissues receive more oxygen and nutrition. The better the circulation of blood around the body, the easier it is to remove the waste products of cells in the body. I don't intend to give a technical explanation of the mechanisms of blood circulation – which is of little interest to the reader who only wishes to lose weight as fat. The bottom line is that with improved circulation and the associated cleansing of cellular waste products *we feel much better.*

And at the end of the day, that's the whole purpose of this diet: to make you look better and feel better.

Now to the exercise 'regime'. There's really no 'regime' at all, and you will be amazed at how easy it is to alter your body shape *medically.* This is really the difference between this programme of exercise and diet, and others that have been published; this is based on established medical principles, whereas some others seem to be little more than the fad of the moment.

First, we have to dispel some common myths about exercise and weight loss:

• *Exercise burns fat*
No, it doesn't! Of course, if you exercise for long periods, it is theoretically possible to burn off fat – but you have to exercise

regularly for extended periods (which is virtually impossible for most people) and it also makes the ridiculous assumption that, after considerable aerobic exercise, you then have the will-power to ignore the ravenous hunger *induced by the exercise*. Perhaps some people can perform this minor miracle, but not many!

• *No pain, no gain*

Absolute rubbish! In fact, worse than rubbish, it's clinically dangerous. If you are overweight and you exercise to the point of inducing pain, the next pain you are likely to experience is that of a coronary thrombosis. In people unaccustomed to regular exercise, exercise must be used only for its primary purpose of toning up the muscles and improving the circulation. This is sufficient to produce a significant improvement in body shape, and actually reduces the risk of a heart attack – with a relatively low level of exercise.

• *You have to exercise for at least an hour per day, three times per week, for it to be effective*

Not true! I will shortly be describing isometric exercises which will tone up your muscles and improve circulation in a few minutes per day. Of course, additional aerobic exercise, in particular walking, is very beneficial. I would advise walking 10–15 minutes per day (which is most easily achieved by either alighting from the bus one stop away from work or parking a little further away).

To exercise properly, you really need to understand a few technical terms. By understanding the *purpose* of what you are doing – which, once again, is very simple – you take control of your own body. Always remember, it's your body, nobody will take as much care of it as you, and armed with the requisite knowledge you can be as healthy as you want to be. The concept of effective exercise is *very* easy, and once you understand the concepts, you will never again be fooled by some of the so-called experts whose only purpose seems to be making a significant proportion of the overweight population feel guilty because they are unable to exercise like Olympic athletes!

Exercise can be **aerobic** or **anaerobic**. **Aerobic** exercise simply means that we take in sufficient oxygen to burn off energy as we exercise. **Anaerobic** exercise is the opposite: we *don't* take in enough oxygen for the exercise, as in sprinting, for example. When you exercise *anaerobically*, your body tells you to stop by giving you pain (from the build-up of a substance called 'lactic acid' in the muscles). So you can now understand why you should **never** experience pain during exercise; it means there is insufficient oxygen for the muscles to perform the exercise in progress. *This is not necessary for effective exercise, in fact it is positively undesirable.*

All of the exercise we perform must be **aerobic**, where we can easily absorb all of the oxygen we need during the activity: in other words, *no pain*. Incidentally, this is *not* the same as *aerobics*, which is just a play on the word 'aerobic'. 'Aerobics' are simply movement exercises, which if too severe may become 'anaerobic' – in other words, they cause pain!

The only other fact you need to know about exercise is that it can be either **isotonic** or **isometric**. This sounds very technical, but it's not; once again, it's very easy to understand. **Isotonic** exercises are those which we immediately think of when the word 'exercise' is mentioned. They involve muscles actually moving: running, lifting, stepping and stretching. In other words, all of the exercises overweight people dislike because they can't do them, and it's embarrassing to try in front of others! The obvious conclusion is that these are *not* the best forms of exercise for the overweight, so isotonic exercises – apart from

walking, which is the best and safest isotonic exercise by far –
are not included in this programme. If you wish, you can
commence isotonic exercises after your muscles have
increased tone and you have lost weight, but it is not essential.

Of course, all forms of exercise – in moderation – can be
beneficial, and if you are currently following a particular exercise
regime, continue that programme. But you should be aware that
jogging and aerobics can be detrimental to knee and hip joints
in those who are significantly overweight, and may have adverse
cardiac (heart) implications if you commence these strenuous
exercises over-enthusiastically for the first time.

The other major category of exercise – which is appropriate
because it can be easily performed by *everyone* – is **isometric**
exercise. In this well-established form of exercise, **muscles do
not move**. That is correct, you exercise *without actually
moving*.

First of all, I tell you that your body fat will *automatically* begin
reducing if you cut out refined carbohydrates from your diet –
but you can eat virtually unlimited amounts of other foods – and
now I am telling you that you can exercise, to become much
stronger and with a significant improvement in body shape –
without moving! No, I haven't lost my senses, and this is true. In
fact, it is a technique routinely used by many athletes in their
training programme.

Isometric exercise is based upon the concept that a muscle
will develop its maximal power *at its resting length*, which
essentially means *without moving but at maximum tension*.

What does that mean in practice? The most effective way to
explain the concept is for you to perform one of these simple
exercises whilst you are sitting reading this book – *but before
commencing any exercise programme, you **must** consult
your doctor first*. Exercising when you are overweight can be
very dangerous unless performed under careful medical

supervision. Isometric exercise can increase blood pressure (and all exercise will increase blood pressure to some degree); therefore **isometric exercise should not be performed by patients with high blood pressure or heart disease.** If you fall into either of these categories, the most beneficial exercise would be walking 10–15 minutes per day.

Providing you have no pre-existing medical condition which is likely to be made worse by unaccustomed exercise, and you have been given the all clear by your doctor, you can proceed with the exercise programme. Remember, you will become slimmer on the diet alone. The exercise programme I am about to describe will merely improve the shape of your slimmer body; it won't actually make you slimmer in itself. So if it's not safe for you to exercise – *don't!* I am first and foremost a physician, which means that I will always advise caution: never take risks with your health!

Let us proceed with an exercise which will clearly demonstrate how easily you can alter your body shape (for the better) in a few minutes per day, and wherever you may be. Place both hands in front of you, elbows bent, palms together, about 15 cm from your chest.

Chest muscle exercise

Now, take a moderate breath in and, whilst holding your breath, press both palms against one another *as hard as you can* for 8–10 seconds, then relax. You have just performed one of the major exercises for strengthening the muscles of the chest (the pectoral muscles). You can probably feel a tightening of the chest muscles already. If you perform this exercise on a daily basis – only 8–10 seconds of continuous exercise – you will strengthen these muscles, and in the process they will assume a smooth contour. As you lose the overlying layer of fat, the body shape underneath will assume a firm, attractive contour, rather than being flabby.

Women need not worry about developing a too muscular body. The beauty of this form of exercise is that it tones muscles but does not create a masculine contour. You will be even more feminine with muscular tone, particularly in 'difficult' areas such as the upper arms. In this part of the female anatomy, excess accumulation of fat cells, in association with poor muscle tone, causes the characteristic appearance of 'dimpled' skin. The diet will reduce the fat layer, and the isometric exercises will increase muscle tone, producing a smoother, firmer upper arm.

Remember, women have a thicker fat layer over their bodies than males, which gives the female form a smoother contour, without muscles 'bulging' out, as in the typical (but rarely seen!) muscular male body shape.

Although this genetically inherited fat layer may seem a disadvantage, it certainly is not; you can use it to your advantage in shaping your body contour. If you diet *properly*, you will retain the underlying muscles, whilst losing some – but not all – of the overlying fat layer. If you then increase the tone of those muscles, their even contour will smooth out the lax overlying skin, removing to a large degree the unsightly dimpling that is sometimes called cellulite.

This rationale works equally successfully for men. You simply use the genetically determined pattern for the shape of your body. What does all this mean? In simple terms, the male body is programmed by its genes to have a thinner fat layer over the muscles than the female. So if you remove the fat, by diet, and increase the tone of the muscles, by isometric exercise, you return to the natural male body shape, with the muscles obvious under a thinner fat layer.

It seems remarkably simple, because it is! The secret is to employ a proper diet and exercise programme to return the body to its natural shape.

If you use the *wrong* diet, and lose protein instead of fat, you will still be thinner, but you cannot then sculpt the body because you don't have any muscles left to sculpt! And if you use the *wrong* exercise programme, you will probably *build* excess muscle, which is often considered unattractive in a woman.

So you can clearly see that correct diet and appropriate exercise will significantly improve body shape *with very little effort or will-power*, and is equally effective in both men and women, because your body is already programmed (through your genes) to assume a particular shape. You are merely returning it to its natural shape by using the *correct* system of exercise and diet.

You can now understand the importance of *effective* dieting. In other words, you reduce *body fat* not *body bulk*: in the former, body protein is saved and body fat is selectively removed, leaving the muscle intact; in the latter, the *size* is reduced, but at the expense of muscle *(or body protein)* rather than *fat*. If planned correctly, an effective diet combined with an appropriate isometric exercise programme will reduce the outer layer of fat and accentuate the underlying muscle.

Of course, we have to exercise *all* of the different muscle groups individually. Our bodies work by having one group of muscles perform one action (for example, moving your leg forward) and another group performing the opposite action (moving the leg backward). If you only exercise the first group, you will become unbalanced in muscular terms, so it is very important that you follow the exercise programme carefully and always exercise *two* groups of muscles on every occasion, the **agonist** and the **antagonist**. Medical terms, but very simple. An 'agonist' is a muscle that moves your body in one direction (for example, bending the arm), and an 'antagonist' is a muscle that moves it in the opposite direction (straightening the arm).

Whenever you exercise an 'agonist' in one direction, you always have to exercise the 'antagonist' muscle in the opposite direction to keep in balance, it's as simple as that. By exercising all of the muscle groups individually, you will achieve an evenly balanced, firm toning of the body, and the whole exercise programme will take no more than 10 minutes per day. These exercises can be performed in the home, at the office or even in the car, whilst waiting in traffic – without you appearing 'odd' to adjacent drivers!

This exercise programme is safer than many others *because you are exercising against yourself*. You are *not* lifting heavy weights, with all the attendant risks involved, or stretching muscles and joints that haven't experienced a wide range of movement for years. In isometric exercise, one half of the body is exercising against the other half, which keeps the body in equal balance, and as you only exert as much effort as you are able, *you* are always in total control of the level of exertion. This is very important because many accidents occur with unaccustomed exercise involving over-exertion with exercise equipment. With isometric exercise, the exercise 'equipment' is your own body!

A comprehensive series of balanced exercises follows. Please follow the recommended exercise programme without omitting any of the exercises, because deviation from the programme could result in an imbalance of muscular power. For example, if you perform the exercise for the front of the arm (to tighten the skin over dimples of cellulite) *without* exercising the rear part of the arm, you will have an imbalance between bending and straightening the arm. Providing you always remember to exercise both the *agonist* muscle and its *antagonist* muscle, which is clearly explained in the table on pages 289–90, you will have no problems.

This daily programme will give you a balanced, toned musculature, in only a little more time than it takes to make a pot of tea!

Chapter 22 An isometric exercise programme

The easiest way of ensuring that you don't miss out any of the main muscle groups when exercising is to start from the head and work down to the toes. Because if you want to look good, your muscle tone has to be balanced from head to foot.

All isometric exercises are performed whilst holding your breath, after inhaling to about half to two-thirds lung capacity, for about 8–10 seconds (the duration of each individual exercise).

The other important point to remember – and I will deliberately repeat this on several occasions because it is very important – is to **take your time** and **rest** during unaccustomed exercise. This whole programme of exercise will take less than four minutes of actual exertion, but I want you to rest for 10–20 seconds between each movement, giving a total time of 10–12 minutes, including resting periods. If you feel uncomfortable at any time, **stop immediately!** Go at your own pace; there is no rush.

Neck exercises

Exercising the neck is *very* important for two main reasons:

1. To help prevent arthritis of the neck

The neck supports the head (fairly obvious), which is mechanically a very difficult action, because the head is relatively heavy and the neck is relatively weak.

Over a period of years, the discs *between* the bones in the neck (vertebrae), gradually wear away at the junctions where the bones rub together.

If you strengthen your neck muscles by isometric exercise you help to prevent arthritis in the neck, which can be very distressing in later life.

2. To improve the cosmetic appearance of the neck

For most people this is the most important reason for exercising the neck. As you know, when you are on a diet there is a tendency for large, unsightly 'craters' to appear in the neck between the muscles where the fat has gone, leaving an undesirable scrawny look. If you simply increase the bulk of the muscle, you will reduce the size of the 'craters', producing a vast improvement in cosmetic appearance.

Isometric neck exercises

The basis of all isometric exercise is that you press *against resistance* for a period of 8–10 seconds. The resistance is provided by other muscles in the body. Neck exercises perform two main movements: forwards/backwards and lateral (side-to-side) movements.

1. Forward/backward isometric neck exercises

Take a deep breath in and hold. Place both hands on the front of your forehead and press your head forwards against your hands as hard as you can.

You should simultaneously press your hands against your forehead, so that there is no movement of your head. Hold this position for 8–10 seconds, then release, breathing in as you relax.

To counterbalance the effect of strengthening these muscles, you must exercise the antagonist group of muscles. Take a deep breath in, place your hands around the back of your head and press your head back against your hands, holding your head motionless by simultaneously pressing forwards with your hands. Hold for 8–10 seconds and release.

2. Lateral isometric neck exercises

Take a deep breath in and hold. Place the palm of your right hand on the right hand side of your head.

Press your head firmly against your hand, resisting the head movement by pressing your hand against your head with equal force. Hold steadily for 8–10 seconds, and release.

Repeat the exercise using the left hand against the left side of the head and hold for 8–10 seconds.

As you can see, these exercises are much harder than you would expect from a contraction of only 8–10 seconds, and you can probably feel the muscle power increasing already.

Isometric chest exercises

We need to exercise the muscles of the upper chest and the corresponding muscles of the upper back because this gives the rounded tone to the upper part of the body that prevents us having a pear-shaped appearance. In a woman these exercises provide tone in the chest musculature under the breasts, giving a slightly increased bust measurement, and, most importantly, an improved *shape* to the bust. However, you will not gain an overly muscular appearance (as normally associated with exercise) because of the slightly thicker overlying fat layer in women.

Place both hands, elbows bent, palms together, approximately 15 cm in front of your chest. Breathe in to about half lung capacity, press both palms together as firmly as you can, hold the contraction for 8–10 seconds whilst holding your breath, and release.

You will feel a tightening of the chest muscles and within a few weeks, these muscles will be much stronger.

As always, we have to balance one group of muscles with their antagonists. The antagonist muscles to the chest are the upper back. To exercise these muscles isometrically, stand with your back to a dining chair (or similar), place both hands behind your back and grasp the respective sides of the chair with both hands.

Take a deep breath in and hold. Press both hands against one another as hard as you can for 8–10 seconds and release, breathing in as you relax.

Isometric upper arm exercises

Toning of the upper arm muscles is cosmetically important for both men and women, for different reasons.

When a woman increases the tone of her muscles, the thicker overlying fat layer ensures a smooth contour to the upper arm, which produces a more cosmetically attractive appearance, removing the undesirable appearance of cellulite. In a man, reduction of the naturally thinner fat layer leads to the desired muscular contour to the biceps. The net result for both sexes is a well-toned upper arm.

We begin by increasing the tone of the *flexor* muscles (biceps). Put your hands by your side. Bend your left arm up to form a right angle, keeping your elbow level with your waist. Your arm should be in a similar position to when you shake someone's hand. Place your right hand over your left wrist and grasp it. Take a deep breath in and hold. Press *up* with your left arm while resisting the movement with your right hand. The left arm should not move during the period of flexion against resistance. Hold the tension for 8–10 seconds, and relax.

Repeat the movement on the right side to exercise the right biceps, once again ensuring that your right elbow stays level with your waist. Your right arm should not move during the exercise.

Obviously, having exercised the *flexor* muscles (biceps) of the arm (which bend it), we have to exercise the *extensor* muscles (triceps) of the arm (which straighten it) to maintain a muscular balance.

Once again, bend your left arm to a right angle, but this time place your right hand *under* your left wrist, before grasping it.

Take a deep breath in and hold. Press *down* with your left arm whilst resisting the movement with your right arm. Hold the tension for 8–10 seconds, and relax.

Repeat the movement on the right side to exercise the right triceps. Hold the tension for 8–10 seconds, and then relax.

Isometric shoulder exercises

The shoulders give the upper body – both male and female – its characteristic shape. The commonest mistake in exercising is to concentrate on the chest and waist, which, although important muscle groups, do not improve the body shape unless you increase shoulder muscle tone. Think about this carefully: if you improve the tone of the shoulder muscles, your posture immediately improves, accentuating the whole body profile. Otherwise, all of your hard work to improve your appearance is undermined by droopy shoulders.

There are several groups of muscles around the shoulder joint, and we can exercise most of them in a total of less than 1 minute!

First, stand in an open doorway and place both hands, palm upwards, against the upper lintel. Take a deep breath in, hold your breath, and press upwards as hard as you can against the upper lintel for 8–10 seconds, then relax and breathe normally. This exercises the muscles on the upper part of the shoulder. Depending on the height of the doorway, you may have to stand on your toes (or possibly a small stool) to reach the lintel, but don't worry, this serves the dual purpose of exercising the muscles on the front of your thigh and the calf at the same time, as they will be in isometric tension during the exercise. You probably never realised how much exercise you could do in 10 seconds without actually moving!

Still standing in the open doorway, make a fist with both hands and place the outer edge of each fist against the sides of the doorway. Take a deep breath in and hold your breath. Press as hard as you can against each door support for 8–10 seconds, and relax. This exercises the muscles on the outer (or lateral) part of the shoulder.

Stand facing a wall, approximately 10 cm away from it. Make a fist with both hands, place the leading edge of both fists against the wall, take a deep breath in and hold your breath. Press as hard as you can against the wall for 8–10 seconds, and relax. This exercises the muscles on the front of the shoulder.

Finally, place your back against the wall, with your shoulders and heels touching the wall. Make a fist with both hands, place the rear edge of both fists against the wall, take a deep breath in and hold, then press back against the wall as hard as you can. Hold the tension for 8–10 seconds and relax. This exercises the muscles on the back of the shoulder.

You can now see that there are many muscle groups around the shoulder that facilitate the complex movements of the arm. We have to exercise all of these groups to maintain stability of the joint. If you exercise some and not others, you will be unbalanced. Within one week of performing these simple – but effective – shoulder muscle exercises you will feel the difference, and the best part of this form of exercising is that the more out of condition you are, the greater the improvement you feel!

Isometric back exercises

One of the major advantages of *isometric* back exercises, rather than the more common *isotonic* exercises, is that they allow you to strengthen your back muscles relatively safely, using only as much resistance as you consider appropriate. **However, anyone with a history of back problems must not commence an exercise programme without the approval of their family physician.**

The first exercise is very important for the latissimus dorsi, a powerful upper back muscle, which also gives a very attractive appearance to the body shape.

Sit on a chair facing a table or desk of normal height, approximately 15 cm away. Place the palms of both hands face down on the table, take a deep breath in and press down as hard as you can on the table whilst holding your breath. Hold the tension for 8–10 seconds, and relax.

The second exercise for the upper back muscles involves using a small towel, such as a tea towel. Stand upright, with feet about shoulder-width apart and your arms holding the towel about shoulder-width apart above your head.

Take a deep breath in and hold. Grasp the towel tightly and try to pull both arms outwards and downwards simultaneously. Hold for 8–10 seconds, and relax.

Isometric exercises for the lower back

The lower back is one of the most important parts of the body for maintaining posture, but it is also one of the main areas of weakness in many people.

Perform all back exercises with extreme caution. If you cannot sustain the contraction for 8–10 seconds, **stop immediately!** Remember, we are solving problems which have gradually developed over decades in many cases. There is *no* rush. You *will* become slimmer, stronger and fitter on the programme, but always *go at your own pace.*

Lie face down on the floor, with your arms by your sides. Take a deep breath in and hold. Raise your head and shoulders about 8–10 cm off the floor, without using your arms. Hold this position for 8–10 seconds, if possible, then relax. You will feel the tension on the lower back muscles, but if there is any discomfort, **stop immediately!**

For the second exercise, lie face down on the carpet, legs and arms extended outwards. Take a deep breath and hold. Arch your back backwards whilst trying to lift your arms and legs off the ground. Hold for 8–10 seconds, and relax.

If you cannot perform this exercise, or perhaps only for a few seconds, don't worry. It is difficult to exercise the back after years of inertia, but as your weight decreases, the exercises *will* become easier, so **do not overexert at this stage**.

Isometric abdominal exercise

Like back exercises, this exercise can cause injuries, because people tend to attack it far too enthusiastically. Remember, the aim is to produce a slimmer, toned and improved body shape, not that of a professional boxer! Only perform the exercise to the level you are able, and that means if you can't do it at this stage, *don't!*

These are exercises that you are not accustomed to, and it would be *abnormal* if you *could* perform the exercises easily. You will look better with a slimmer waist from the diet, and as the fat decreases you will gradually be able to perform the abdominal exercise with ease. Do what you can, no more, and *never be afraid to stop*. No pain, no gain is for fools!

Lie flat on your back with your hands by your sides. Take a deep breath and hold, then gently lift the upper part of your body about 10 cm off the ground (using your abdominal muscles; don't push up with your hands) and hold for 8–10 seconds (or less), then relax. This is all you need to do to tighten your abdominal muscles and improve abdominal shape, *but it is a hard exercise in the beginning, so do not over-exert yourself.*

Isometric leg exercises

Isometric exercises for the leg muscles are relatively easy to perform, and have the added advantage that several groups of muscles can be exercised in the same movement.

The first exercise involves standing in an open doorframe, with your back resting against one doorpost. Lift one leg and place the foot against the other doorpost at a height that is convenient to you; in other words, don't try to lift your leg high if it is not comfortable. Take a deep breath in and hold your breath. Brace your back against the doorpost and press against the other doorpost as hard as you can for 8–10 seconds, then relax. Repeat the exercise with the other leg.

This is an excellent exercise for toning up the muscles on the front of the thigh (quadriceps) and also the all-important calf muscles, which give the lower leg its contour.

Having exercised the muscles on the front of the leg, we now have to exercise the rear of the leg (the hamstring muscles) and the muscles on the bottom. Toning this area is essential, as I am sure all will agree.

Stand with your back to a wall, both heels and shoulders resting against the wall. Place the palms of both hands flat against the wall for stability. Take a deep breath in and hold, then press your right heel as hard as you can against the wall – without propelling yourself forward – for 8–10 seconds, and relax. You will feel the tightening of the muscles down the back of your leg, and especially the buttock region, almost immediately.

Repeat the exercise with the left leg.

That completes the programme. Of course, I could describe isometric exercises that would improve the tone and strength of virtually every muscle group in the body, but that is not the purpose of this book. The purpose is to show you how to tone the most important muscle groups, to ensure an attractive, contoured body after removing the surface layer of fat with effective dieting. This requires only 23 exercises, each of 8–10 seconds' duration, a total of 4 minutes of actual exercise. Allowing for a resting period of 20 seconds between each movement – which is double the exercise duration itself – the total time required is a maximum of 12 minutes per day. The exercises are briefly summarised in the following table.

Isometric exercise programme

	Agonist	**Antagonist**
1. **Neck**	forward movement (flexion)	backward movement (extension)
	movement to right side	movement to left side
2. **Thorax**	chest muscles	upper back muscles
3. **Shoulder**	arm movement forwards	arm movement backwards
	arm movement up	arm movement down
4. **Upper arm**	bending (flexion)	straightening (extension)

5. **Upper back**	arm movement	arm movement
	up	down
6. **Abdomen**	abdominal	lower back
	muscles	muscles
7. **Leg**	front leg muscles	rear leg muscles
	(quadriceps)	(hamstrings and
		calf muscles)

I must emphasise that it is essential to *take it easy* when you start exercising. This programme is ideal because it is relatively easy, can be taken at your own pace, requires no special equipment and is highly effective in achieving results, but I still advise you to take your time. If you feel uncomfortable, *stop!* Remember you are still losing weight on the diet, and there is no desperate rush to increase muscle tone. Exercise must achieve its aims *gently* to be safe and effective.

At this point, it would be useful to review what this exercise programme will achieve, and also what it will not!

- If you don't diet to lose the fat, the muscles will be toned, but you won't notice them through the overlying fat layer. The exercise in itself will *not* cause significant loss of fat – but then that was never the intention.
- If you diet incorrectly, and lose protein as well as fat, you will not be able to achieve a toned body, because there is very little muscle to tone, so an appropriate *fat-losing* (not just weight-losing), *muscle-sparing* diet is essential. A high-protein, low-carbohydrate diet will achieve this desired result.
- Isometric exercise will tone and strengthen the body musculature, giving a more attractive body shape. It won't increase stamina, which can only be achieved by repetitive, time-consuming isotonic exercises (such as

using a treadmill), but then you don't really need this for most of the time. If you lose fat and increase body protein, you will feel better and have more energy anyway! If you can combine these isometric exercises with a little walking (10–15 minutes per day) or swimming, you will notice a substantial improvement in your fitness level. Remember, 10–15 minutes' walking is only 10 minutes to and from the bus stop or to your car, every day. It requires virtually no special arrangements or equipment to achieve. And it is medically proven to reduce risks of heart attack significantly.

Exercise of any form, especially when combined with an appropriate diet, will change your shape, but it will not attain the impossible. Be realistic and have realistic goals. Having lost all the *unnecessary* weight (as fat) and toned your muscles, you will look and feel immensely better, but it will still be you. Don't try to be someone else. The supermodels in magazines have the advantage of a photographer with an air-brush to remove any presumed cosmetic defects; it's not real life, and they don't look like that in real life!

Appendix 1

The carbohydrate content of common snack foods

i. Foods which may be included in the diet within the 40-gram daily carbohydrate limit, with extreme caution

(Some of these items vary in size and ingredients; the carbohydrate contents are average values and can vary)

Food	Average carbohydrate content (grams of carbohydrate)
Biscuits (per biscuit)	
bourbon	8
chocolate chip	7
chocolate coated	12
cream	7
crunch cream	9
custard cream	8
digestive	
– chocolate	11
– plain	11
ginger nut	9
shortbread	11
Crackers and crispbreads (per cracker/crispbread)	
catcakes	6
cream cracker	5
rye crispbread	6
water biscuit	5
wholemeal cracker	5

Fruit
(per piece)

apple	13
grapefruit	10
grapes (100g)	14
kiwi fruit	10
mango (half)	12
melon (honeydew)	11
nectarine	7
orange	10
peach	9
plum	9

Nuts
(per 100g)

almond	2
Brazil	3
hazelnuts	6
macadamia	5
peanuts	12
pecan	6
pine	4
pistachio	8
walnut	3

Potato crisps
(per bag)

bacon and brown sauce	12
roast beef	12
roast chicken	12
tomato	12
salt	12
salt and vinegar	11
sour cream and onion	14

ii. Foods which should *not* be included in the diet
(These items vary in size and ingredients; the carbohydrate contents are average values and can vary)

Food	Average carbohydrate content (grams of carbohydrate)
Bread (each)	
bagel	30
focaccia	30
pitta	55
roll	29
sliced	15–17 (maximum of 1 slice/day)
tortilla	20–25 (maximum of 1/day)
Cake (per 100g)	
apple pie	30
banana	62
cheesecake	30
chocolate	55
chocolate éclair	30
Danish pastry	42
doughnut	40
fruit	55
muffin	50
scone	46
sponge	50

Cereal
(per 100g)
(examples only – *all* breakfast cereals are excluded)

muesli	72
puffed wheat	65
sultana bran	66

Fast food
(per 100g)
bacon and egg
  muffin

per muffin	33
cheeseburger	
per burger	35
chicken dippers	
per dipper	2
chicken nuggets	
per nugget	3
chicken, fried	
per piece (approx)	45

chips
(oven-bake)

per portion	72
hash brown	
per piece	15
onion bhajia	
per bhajia	4

pizza (per 100g)
  (varies)

average pizza	33
per slice	25
examples:	
cheese and tomato	
(deep pan)	45
cheese and tomato	
(thin and crispy)	28

four cheese (thin and crispy)	32
vegetable and goat's cheese (thin and crispy)	31
potato wedges (oven-bake)	25
Quarter Pounder	20
saffron rice	24
sausage roll	25
per roll	30
shepherd's pie (beef, per 100g)	10
pie (lamb, per 100g)	11
spring roll per roll	50
vegetable pakora	20
vegetable samosa	25
Fruit banana	30
pear	19
Ice cream (100 ml)	20
Milk chocolate (per 100g)	61
Mixed nuts and raisins (per 100g)	32

Appendix 2 The carbohydrate content of vegetables

i. Vegetables included without restriction in the diet

Vegetable (100g)	Average carbohydrate content (grams of carbohydrate)
Asparagus (fresh)	2
Aubergine	2
Avocado	2
Bamboo shoots	6
Beans (French)	3
Broccoli	1
Brussels sprouts	2
Cabbage	2
Carrots	7
Cauliflower	2
Celery	2
Courgettes	2
Cucumber	3
Garlic (per clove)	less than 1
Kale	5
Lettuce	2
Mushrooms (button)	2
Onions	4
Parsley	less than 1
Peas	7
Peppers:	
green	2.5
red	4
yellow	4
Pumpkin	7
Radish	2

Spinach	1
Tomatoes	3
Turnips	2
Swede	2

ii. Vegetables excluded from the diet during the weight-loss phase

Vegetable (100g)	Average carbohydrate content (grams of carbohydrate)
Beetroot	14
Chickpeas	16
Corn (cob)	12
Haricot beans	18
Kidney beans	12
Lentils	17
Parsnips	13
Potatoes	
boiled	14
chipped	36
Sweet potato	21
Yam	38

Appendix **3** The carbohydrate content of alcoholic beverages

Beverage	Average carbohydrate content (grams of carbohydrate)
Beer (1 pint)	13
Sherry (50 ml)	
dry	less than 1
sweet	4
Spirits (50 ml)	
brandy	0
gin	0
vodka	0
whisky	0
Wine (100 ml)	
red	less than 1
white	
dry	less than 1
medium	4
sweet	6

Index

RECIPES

BREAKFAST
Baked haddock with grilled Swiss
    cheese 76
Blueberries with mixed nuts and

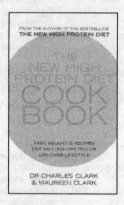

**Also available from Vermilion by
Dr Charles Clark and Maureen Clark**

THE HEALTHY LOW GI LOW CARB DIET

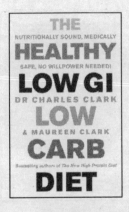

The revolutionary low carb dietary phenomenon continues to attract an enormous following. Yet for many it is not an option. Dr Charles Clark has devised a low-carb, low GI plan that caters for all types of dietary requirement, including vegetarians, who cannot follow a plan with high-meat content, and those who need natural fibre in their diet. It's vegetarian-friendly and nutritionally balanced, allowing for previously sinful foods including pasta, pulses, fruit and puddings. What's more, he has set out to counter the criticisms of those who argue that low-carb lifestyles can be detrimental to health and reveals how adopting a low-carbohydrate diet can in fact be of benefit in certain key areas of health.

£8.99   ISBN 9780091902544

Order direct from www.rbooks.co.uk/charlesclark

**Also available from Vermilion by
Dr Charles Clark and Maureen Clark**

THE ULTIMATE DIET COUNTER

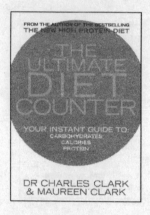

Featuring over 3,000 listings, this food counter is organised
into sensible food groups and provides just the right level of
information for a quick look-up. It's the perfect guide to keep in
your bag as a handy companion to any diet, enabling you to
look up any food and work out whether it's going to work on
your diet, whether it's calorie controlled, low-carb or low-fat.

£3.99   ISBN 9780091889715

Order direct from www.rbooks.co.uk/charlesclark